Nick Stafford

Kindly Donated
by
Dr Stafford

THE INNER APPRENTICE

DEDICATION

In gratitude to the memory of the late
Frank Thomas,
an inspirational schoolmaster.
A teacher of classics, divinity and music,
more by vision than by accomplishment
he enlarged the lives of
countless pupils and friends.

THE INNER APPRENTICE

APPRENTICE

**An awareness–centred approach
to Vocational Training for General Practice**

ROGER NEIGHBOUR

MA, MB, BChir, DObstRCOG, FRCGP

General Practitioner, Abbots Langley, Hertfordshire

Trainer and past Course Organiser,
Watford Vocational Training Scheme

1988 Fellow of
The Association of Course Organisers

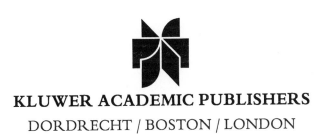

KLUWER ACADEMIC PUBLISHERS
DORDRECHT / BOSTON / LONDON

Also by Roger Neighbour: *The Inner Consultation – How to develop and effective and intuitive consulting style.* Kluwer; 1987 (reprinted 4 times). ISBN 0-7462-0040-4

Distributors

for the United States and Canada: Kluwer Academic Publishers, PO Box 358, Accord Station, Hingham, MA 02018-0358, USA

for all other countries: Kluwer Academic Publishers Group, Distribution Center, PO Box 322, 3300 AH Dordrecht, The Netherlands

British Library Cataloguing in Publication Data

A catalogue record for this book is available from the British Library.

Library of Congress Cataloging-in-Publication Data

Neighbour, Roger, 1947–
    The inner apprentice : an awareness-centered approach to vocational training for general practice / Roger Neighbour.
       p.   cm.
    Includes bibliographical references.
    ISBN 0-7923-8983-2 (casebound)
    1. Medicine—Study and teaching (Continuing education) I. Title.
    [DNLM: 1. Education, Medical, Continuing. 2. Teaching—methods.
W 20 N397i]
    R737.N45   1992
    610'.0071'5—dc20
    DNLM/DLC
    for Library of Congress   92-2938
                                                        CIP

Copyright

Published in the United Kingdom by Kluwer Academic Publishers, PO Box 55, Lancaster.

Kluwer Academic Publishers BV incorporates the publishing programmes of D. Reidel, Martinus Nijhoff, Dr W. Junk and MTP Press.

Printed and bound in Great Britain by Butler and Tanner Ltd., Frome and London.

Contents

Chapter 9: The Inner Curriculum   **182**

References and Bibliography   **219**

Foreword

Throughout the 1970s and 1980s those involved in vocational training for general practice have spent much time, and expended considerable energy, in refining systems and methods for teaching trainees. As a result, lists of content have been agreed, appropriate teaching methods have been defined and ways for assessing progress have been formulated. This has given teachers a greater confidence in their ability to teach and learners a clearer idea of what is expected of them. Nevertheless, most would acknowledge that there is considerably more to be done to improve the quality of education available to individual young doctors. The less definable yet important areas of practice remain elusive and difficult to address through the training systems that have been developed. A key is needed that will open up the more attitudinal areas of practice and of training. There can be no better person to fashion such a key than Roger Neighbour.

As the first Fellow appointed by the Association of Course Organisers in 1988, Roger Neighbour undertook a survey to try to distinguish the characteristics of trainees considered outstanding from those who did not reach their full potential. From this work he was able to formulate fourteen hallmarks of excellence in trainee general practitioners. These are presented in *The Inner Apprentice*, which goes on to consider how these hallmarks can be inculcated through a broader range of educational strategies than those currently deployed in vocational training. By shifting the focus from how teachers teach to the other side of the educational equation — how people learn — Roger Neighbour enables us to understand what previously had been undefinable.

Learning is an inborn ability that cannot be suppressed. *The Inner Apprentice* explores the role of the teacher in the learning process and demonstrates how changes in balance between teacher and learner can influence learning itself. It draws on examples from the philosophers and legends of Ancient Greece, from the apprentice-masters of medieval Europe, from the fiction of modern literature and films and from the sportsmen of today to illuminate with clarity the philosophy and principles that can enhance the learning process. The book introduces the concept of awareness-based teaching and shows how specific awareness-raising techniques can widen the scope of what people learn, particularly in the softer and more attitudinal areas of the individual that include self-awareness, motivation, compassion and industry.

Roger Neighbour's first book, *The Inner Consultation*, was widely and deservedly praised for its new perspective on this essential part of practice. What this book did for the doctor/patient relationship, *The Inner Apprentice* will do for the trainer/trainee relationship through exploration of the less explicit levels of communication between teacher and learner. Roger Neighbour has first-hand experience of the difficulties that young doctors encounter in practice and in training through his work as an MRCGP examiner, as a trainer, and as a former Course Organiser. He makes readily understandable a series of profound ideas by using illustrations that range from Socrates through *The Karate Kid* to the consulting room itself. His book will help to eliminate what hitherto has been a black hole in vocational training, and will provide insights into the intricacies and tensions of the trainer/trainee relationship so that the interaction embodied in it can be put to best educational effect. It will refresh and re-energise those who are established in the field; it will enthuse and inspire those who are new to training; and cannot fail to entertain and inform all who read it.

Bill Styles
Chairman, Education Division,
Royal College of General Practitioners;
Regional Adviser in General Practice,
North West Thames Region

Acknowledgements

Pre-eminent amongst those to whom I owe an immeasurable debt is the Association of Course Organisers. They did me the great honour of electing me in 1988 to their first Fellowship, and commissioned the study of the 'Hallmarks of Excellence' described in Chapter 3. Britain's doctors and patients have more to thank the Course Organisers for than they often realise. It is largely through their devotion to the values of academic rigour and innovation, and to their enthusiasm and resilience, that vocation is so often transmuted into good practical patient care. I thank them for their generosity of spirit and funds.

Nearer home, I appreciate the common sense and gentle wisdom of my friends in the Watford Vocational Training Scheme Trainers' Workshop, especially its leader Dr Peter Bennett.

Like all Trainers, I am constantly reminded of being reciprocally apprenticed to my own Trainees. In recent years Graham and Glyn and Tim and Dominic have given lavishly of their stimulating curiosity.

To Dr Bill Styles, who has written the Foreword to this and my previous book, I want to say "Thank you" for many instances of support and permission-giving at various stages of both our careers. He has been to me a more valued mentor than I have ever told him to his face.

In the course of developing the ideas presented here I have enjoyed meeting some unique talents, especially those of the sociologist Professor Stephen Cotgrove, the athlete David Hemery, the sports coach Alan Fine, and the educational psychologist Peter Honey. I wish medicine could teach other disciplines half as much as they can teach it.

It's hard to recall all the people who have said the right thing at the right time. But I do know that discussion with Timothy Gallwey, author of *The Inner Game* books, set me thinking years back about how we can improve our performance of complex tasks; that Dr Ken Burch introduced me to

Roger Lipsey's pearl-in-the-oyster piece on medieval apprenticeship; and Dr John Charlewood told me the Arabic proverb about pupils and teachers quoted hereafter.

I am grateful for the following permissions to quote from published works:

An Art of Our Own by Roger Lipsey; © 1988 by Roger Lipsey. Reprinted by arrangement with Shambala Publications, Inc., 300 Massachusetts Ave., Boston, MA 02115, USA.

Mutative Metaphors in Psychotherapy: the Aeolian Mode, by Murray Cox and Alice Theilgaard; © 1987 by Murray Cox and Alice Theilgaard. Reprinted by kind permission of Tavistock Publications.

Between Psychology and Psychotherapy: A Poetics of Experience, by Miller Mair; © 1989 by Miller Mair. Reprinted by kind permission of Routledge.

Sexist pronouns

These days, when a person writes a book he or she has to agonize over how they are going to overcome one's pronoun problem. A man-as-opposed-to-monkey doesn't know what s/he should do for the best. Anyway, I'm a male Trainer. Most of the Trainers I know are male. So in this book Trainers get male pronouns. Trainees do too, sometimes; but not always. Not when they're female. Now I do understand that, in books as on buses and trains, women don't like 'men' to stand for them any more. But then, sometimes they don't mind. Sorry if anyone's upset. Blame the English language. It isn't my fault. Or one's. Or his/hers. Or theirs. Or men's-as-opposed-to-women's. It's its.

He that knows not,
　　and knows not that he knows not,
　　　　is a fool.
　　　　　　Shun him.

He that knows not,
　　and knows that he knows not,
　　　　is a pupil.
　　　　　　Teach him.

He that knows,
　　and knows not that he knows,
　　　　is asleep.
　　　　　　Wake him.

He that knows,
　　and knows that he knows,
　　　　is a teacher.
　　　　　　Follow him.

(Arabic proverb)

Part I
On Apprenticeship

During my childhood – I slept in bed.
During my adolescence – I waited at the door.
In my maturity – I have flown towards the heavens!

Constantin Brancusi

Chapter 1
On apprenticeship

INTRODUCTION

Mankind creates an institution out of every instinct. And around every cultural institution an invisible wall is built, to separate a favoured group of insiders from the envious also-rans on the outside.

Things seem to have been this way throughout history. Once upon a time, Adam falls in love with Eve, and lo! – the world has had wedlock ever since. One day Adam stumbles and hurts himself, and hey presto! – health professionals. He turns to Eve for comfort, and before long the Earth teems with duly accredited psychotherapists. They peer curiously at the natural world about them, and the foundation stones of Universities are laid. Huddled anxiously beside an uncertain fire they gaze up at the stars and ask the unanswerable questions; and in their disputing is foreshadowed the Inquisition. They divert each other with stories, anticipating Hollywood. Their sons Cain and Abel fall out; posterity clamours at the doors of its Law Courts and Child Guidance Clinics. The grandchildren play 'I'm the king of the castle'; nowadays the more gentle of their descendants compete in the Olympics, while the rougher ones stand for Parliament.

Learning too is instinctive. A person can't *not* learn. For better or worse, humankind's impact on the planet would be insignificant were it not that the acquired experience of each generation can be bequeathed to the very next. To learn is to accelerate evolution. However, the instinct to learn is also matched by an irresistible urge to interfere. Every society festoons the curiosity of its youngsters with the trappings of institutionalised control. 'To learn' is *one* thing, as natural as digesting or drawing breath. 'To educate' is quite another. 'Education' implies teacher as well as pupil, active and passive, donor and recipient. 'Education' implies curriculum, syllabus, assessment, sanctions. Seemingly it calls for expertise and theory, for enormous investment in man-power and resources, and, above all, for effort.

In the 1970s the philosopher Ivan Illich published a series of diatribes against the professions – law, medicine, education, management, religion [1]*. His theme was a variation on the conspiracy theory of history. Shrieking "incompetence" and "plot", he accused the professions of cornering the market in human vulnerability and conspiring to exploit the ordinary needs of ordinary folk. In submitting to this subjugation, Illich contended, people's natural coping abilities withered and died. I can't help wondering whether Illich might not have been right (well, right-ish), but for the wrong reason.

My own field, General Practice, encompasses so many scientific and liberal disciplines that it seems unavoidable, if aspiring GPs are to have any career time left to practise, for their learning to take place within an agreed organisational and conceptual tradition. Vocational Training for General Practice in Great Britain has a short but proud tradition of administrative systems and theoretical constructs, and an admirable teaching network of skilled and generous enthusiasts. And for what, if not to help Trainees by shortening and intensifying the period it takes to become competent? I dare say the same is true as well for most other areas of postgraduate and professional training. What is tradition, after all, if not history's arm around the shoulders of the present generation?

But do things turn out as intended? It has to be admitted that Vocational Training doesn't always seem to succeed in direct proportion to the goodwill of its Trainers. I suspect the reason is that the complexity and rigidity of some of the educational methods we've come to take for granted are beginning, like grit within a bearing, to hinder the smooth running of the very enterprise they're intended to lubricate. We teachers do our very best. We want, quite unashamedly, the very best for our Trainees. We combine educational theory with common sense and sensitivity as well as we can. We try to be systematic and diligent. Very often our pupils are responsive, and this gives us well-deserved satisfaction. But not always. Not often enough. Some Trainees don't respond to educational strategies which have succeeded with others. They become our disappointments and frustrations. We feel we have let them down, but we may not know how. And at such times the usual lament, "But I did everything I was supposed to", comes as little consolation.

It's not for one moment my intention to decry all the paraphernalia of formal postgraduate education. In the course of my own career, Vocational Training in General Practice has served me well, and I love being part of it. However – in occupations where kindness and concern are professional virtues, and as the educational intricacies proliferate – it's my

---

* Numbers in square brackets refer to entries in the References and Bibliography, p.219.

belief that something vital is in danger of being lost sight of. This book is about what that mysterious ingredient might be: for now, let's call it 'the personal touch'.

THE 'DEEP STRUCTURE' AND 'SURFACE STRUCTURE' OF EDUCATIONAL SYSTEMS

I want for a moment to look beneath the surface features of our postgraduate educational institutions: to concentrate, as it were, less on their facial expressions and more on the underlying bone structure.

Many areas of human experience are so commonplace and yet at the same time so important and so complex that we tend to communicate about them in a kind of code. Politics, morality and personal relationships are examples of fields where, time being short and total honesty being risky, we conduct our business in shorthand. We simplify the complexity of our true thoughts and feelings into a series of reach-me-down responses, slogans and stylized expressions, and transact our affairs using these tokens for currency. Most of our utterances about important topics are less than complete representations of what we *could* express, did we but choose to. And most of the time this process of being 'economical with the truth' is good enough. In spite of what we say, people usually know what we mean. As long as we all take the same things for granted, we all get by.

Linguistics – the study of meaning as expressed in words – draws an important distinction, which will help us now, between the 'surface structure' of a person's speech and the 'deep structure' of which it is an incomplete expression [2]. If I say to you, "Education is a good thing", you will probably agree; how could you not? The *reason* you will agree has as much to do with *your* assumptions about what *I* mean, and the extent to which *your* assumptions coincide with what you *believe* mine to be, as it does with any intrinsic truth my assertion might possess. The sentence, "Education is a good thing", is impeccable English syntax, and to that extent is perfectly comprehensible. But it leaves unanswered a number of questions which are vital if your agreement is to have any value. What, for instance, do I mean by "education"? University places for all who desire them, or the brain-washing of social dissidents? And what does "good" mean in this context? Cost-effective? Salutary? Fun? Good for whom? And if education is good, what would I consider bad by comparison? All these points and many others would have to be clarified if you were fully to understand my remark's deep structure. It would have to be freed from its assumptions and value-judgements, and a great deal of detail added, before you could know whether or not it was truly acceptable to you.

Life's too short. Most of the time we don't bother to retrieve the deep structure of every communication from its surface representation. We make do with an inference. The surface structure will do to get by with. And yet the deep structure's meaning may, for all we know, be something quite different – something to which, did we but fully comprehend it, we might respond differently.

We can be equally unquestioning of our educational system and its methodology. Educational systems have 'surface structures', such as timetables, curricula, schools, teachers and examinations. They also have 'deep structures' – philosophical assumptions about what ought to be taught, and who ought to be taught it, and how, as well as more subversive issues about the division of power, control and accountability between teachers and pupils. Specifically, we *think* we know what postgraduate educational programmes are striving to achieve, (and those who organise them probably *think* they know as well). But it might be timely, without decrying their motives, to examine some of their underlying assumptions and principles. Perhaps we might question the conclusion that, because teachers are well-intentioned people, the deep structures they serve are equally benevolent.

It is possible to discern two quite distinct but co-existent deep structures represented in today's educational orthodoxy. Each has a perfectly valid historical pedigree, and each has made a distinctive contribution to the educational surface structures we currently take for granted. I want to discriminate between the two, for my contention developed in this book is that we are in danger of emphasising one too exclusively at the expense of the other. One deep structure – the more predominant at the moment – I'll call 'education as *Revelation*'. A second is 'education as *Quest*'. (And I further want to suggest that there is a third deep structure which we would do well to resurrect from its historical antecedents. This will be 'education as *Apprenticeship*'.)

Education as 'Revelation'

A great deal of contemporary education is similar in deep structure to the revelation of the ten commandments to the Israelites – the law vouchsafed from God to the masses, with a prophet acting as go-between. You remember the story. The Hebrews, after escaping the bondage of the Egyptian Pharaohs and wandering aimlessly in the wilderness, seemed to Moses their leader to be in need of guidance. Moses climbed Mount Sinai, the scene of his own original calling, where (if Hollywood is to be believed) God with a display of special effects spelt out life's core curriculum on tablets of stone. The returning prophet found that while his back had been turned the rank and file had forgotten even the little morality they *had* known, and were into freedom of expression in a big way. Moses in temper smashed the stone tablets and had to go back for a second copy. Cowed by Jehovah's threat not to sign their Statements of Satisfactory Completion, the Israelites learned the ten commandments by heart and lived chosen ever after.

This story is clearly a metaphor for the more didactic of today's educational methods. Most teachers, myself included, will acknowledge the seductiveness of the teacher's Mosaic role as mouthpiece for the Almighty. But this 'education as a process of revelation' is predicated on a number of assumptions – a deep structure – which when starkly presented demand reappraisal. The assumptions are:

(1) There exists a body of knowledge which is finite, valuable, eternal, and (in some ultimate sense) true.

(2) The task of education is to transfer this received wisdom intact and uncorrupted into the minds of those previously ignorant of it.

(3) The role of the teacher is to have acquired expertise by prior preparation, and to possess sufficient skill or charisma to overcome the pupil's innate ignorance.

(4) The pupil's natural tendency is to misunderstand what he is told: the best safeguard against this is a clearly defined system of curriculum and assessment which will identify any shortcomings in learning and allow their correction.

(5) Left to their own devices, pupils will probably make ill-informed and inappropriate choices about what and how they prefer to learn: pupils' autonomy is perceived as a threat to reliability – something than can, if necessary, be sacrificed on the altar of curriculum.

It's not difficult to recognise in this admittedly rather overstated description the educational shortcomings of which traditional hospital-based medical teaching is rightly accused. And we can all claim, like Calvin Coolidge's preacher on the subject of sin, that we are against it. Yet it remains widespread. Either we are blind and helpless before its power, or it else has hidden attractions: probably the latter. I think the attraction of didactic teaching lies in the belief (shared by teacher and pupil alike, though for different reasons) that the impetus to learn is supplied from *outside* the learner. Perceiving the 'locus of opportunity' as external absolves the pupil of blame if he fails to learn, and at the same time affords the teacher the illusion of glory if the learning goes well.

Within any discipline that requires its initiates to achieve mastery of a defined body of knowledge, the role of an educational system, like that of sex in the biological field, is to reproduce its kind. The trouble is, with an externally-located source of instruction it's all but impossible to transmit the necessary content without at the same time transmitting the deep structure's message that 'Teacher knows best'. Along with the heirloom of knowledge and skill, the pupil also inherits passivity of mind, subservience and unoriginality. This is a hard legacy to be rid of.

Where it is considered important for the next intellectual generation to resemble its predecessors; and when, therefore, it is necessary to procreate mechanisms of cognitive and cultural control to maintain the status quo, then a dogmatic educational style is appropriate. But, whatever other virtues they may have as academic touchstones, curriculum and assessment are also the twin gonads of conservatism. Dogma inspires few dreams; and without dreams, what use is freedom?

Education as 'Quest'

The other current contender for the educational high ground believes that the 'locus of opportunity' lies *within* the learner, who possesses an intrinsic drive for self-fulfilment. Moreover, it maintains, everything that needs to be known the pupil at some level already knows: what he has to do is to discover it. The teacher's role consists of setting up the circumstances in which productive introspection can occur. This is 'education as Quest'. There are close similarities between this educational style and the process of non-directive counselling, a comparison which to the new wave of teachers is a flattering one.

Good examples of education as Quest, sufficiently unfamiliar to allow critical appraisal, are to be found in the training of neophytes in many religious traditions. This is how novices undertaking training in the Zen school of Buddhism are led towards their own personal realisation [3].

A postulant seeking admission to a training monastery faces a series of daunting ordeals. On arrival he is told to go away: the monastery is full; he is not the right 'type'; his credentials are not satisfactory. The poor chap is kept waiting in the entrance hall for three days and nights, during which time he remains crouched over his few belongings, except at those times when he is physically ejected for an hour at a time. Yet this is not wanton or arbitrary unkindness – it is already the beginning of the training the novice seeks. Awe of the unfamiliar is considered a necessary prerequisite for the radical refashioning in store. The head training monk would explain, "If you really want to come in, you must leave your self outside, and then you will have no difficulty in the training. But if you take your previous self inside, you will have nothing but difficulties yourself, and make difficulties for the community."

The early months of Zen training are structured to help the Trainee make the transition from his previous assumptions and priorities and instead to redirect his expectations towards an experiential way of learning. He is set the most menial tasks, and is given no instruction in how to perform them, beyond the cursory advice to keep his eyes open. The Master is revered as an example of what may be attained, but he won't explain. Instead the monk learns through meditation to look within himself for the source of his transformation. In his personal interviews with the Master, he is confronted with seemingly crazy and impenetrable conundrums which wrestle agonizingly with his intellect. Producing his ceremonial staff, the Master may say, "If you call this a stick it is disgusting; if you say it is not a stick you are in error. What will you call it?" Whatever the pupil says seems to be wrong. Today's answer is never the 'right' one, even though tomorrow it may have been. Near the end of his tether, he can't tell what is valuable and what is not. And yet this is the whole point, for just *beyond* the end of his tether is the enlightenment he had been seeking. Encompassing all this apparent turmoil is a tradition that knows that when a person is emptied of all previous certainty, and forced to look nowhere other than within for a replacement, insight of the most profound kind can emerge self-generated and self-transcendent.

There is clearly much in common between the deep structures of the Zen way of training and our own Vocational Training system. Come to think of it, their surface structures are fairly similar also: the ordeal of the selection process to get accepted onto a scheme; the promise of mysteries to be revealed only when previous habits of mind are un-learned; the balance between service commitment, small group work and one-to-one tutorials; the Trainer who is at once slave driver, sonofabitch and Saint.

As we did when considering the 'revelatory' style, let us examine the assumptions made by the deep structure of the 'quest' model. They include:

(1) Knowledge that 'really' matters – the wisdom that endures and is transferable to every situation – is already latent in the pupil from the outset; specific details can be acquired from the environment by a process of osmosis to which not much attention need be paid.

(2) The task of education is to provide an environment in which the pupil's capacity for self-transformation can be realised, and self-selected goals accomplished.

(3) The role of the teacher is that of facilitator, not provider; a good teacher structures the pupil's experience over time, presenting the pupil with a succession of challenges to entice the expansion of his innate abilities. The teacher complements this process with the ability to support, sustain and motivate.

(4) The pupil's natural state is curiosity: he senses, however subliminally at first, his own needs, and will in time satisfy them without extraneous constraints.

(5) Left to themselves, however, pupils tend to look for short-cuts in the form of instruction from 'experts'. This inertia is perceived as a threat to true fulfilment, and something to be dispelled by a resolutely heuristic teaching style.

This style of teaching is all the rage in Vocational Training for General Practice at the moment. Approval is signalled by phrases like 'Trainee-centred' and 'self-directed learning'. It is capable of extremely rewarding results and attracts many genuine enthusiasts. And almost every Trainer pays it lip-service. But why sometimes only lip-service?

The trouble with having the 'locus of opportunity' within the pupil is that as teachers we can't directly get at it. The ability to motivate appears to be one of the most important qualities a teacher needs to possess, and we don't know how to do this – not reliably, at any rate. An effective piece of heuristic teaching is likely to draw little applause for the teacher, the Trainee being rightly credited. If on the other hand a Trainee systematically underachieves within this model, we teachers wring our hands in guilt over our inadequacies as facilitators of self-directed learning. Then we might ask ourselves just how a person is supposed to *know* what he's capable of achieving, unless someone didactically gives a clue. With returning confidence we assert that, while discovery is all very well and can doubtless be very effective, it may not be the universal panacea. In some circumstances, surely, *telling* can be quicker, more efficient and less frustrating for both parties.

Agreed. In their pure forms, 'Revelation' and 'Quest' have their shortcomings. So what's to be done? The traditional British compromise? A bit of each, pick and mix? It's tempting to reach for the clichés – "horses for courses", "seat of the pants".

'Process' and 'trajectory'

Let's instead see if we can't feel the arm of history reassuringly around our shoulders. Two arms of history, in fact. The first is from Classical Greece. The educational legacy of Socrates – his preposterous skill at leading people by the nose towards the truth – is far from being exhausted. From Socrates we can learn how, by the judicious timing and structuring of our awareness-raising questions, to manage an effective educational encounter on a moment-by-moment time-scale. In today's jargon, Socrates can teach us *process*. The second is from Medieval Europe, where the guilds of craftsmen developed the most marvellous system of training by apprenticeship which can stand today as a template for our own attempts. Medieval apprenticeship, like the more arcane training of the Zen novice described earlier, was uniquely successful because the craftmasters were able to structure the experience of their apprentices and journeymen over weeks and months into an overall calendar of maturation. The vocabulary of Vocational Training has hitherto lacked a word (and perhaps, therefore, a concept) to describe this sequencing of the various educational components, their inter-relationships and psychodynamics, over the course of an extended traineeship. It's not mere 'content', and it's more than what we usually mean by 'process'. I propose the term 'trajectory': it has the right associations of a launching-point, a progress through the sky towards a chosen target, and a sense of movement through time and space. The medieval craftsmen can teach us the importance of guiding the *trajectory* of a traineeship.

SOCRATES

"An unquestioned life is not worth living."

Carry your imagination to Athens – not today's clogged and corroded ant-hill, but the Athens of five centuries before Christ: the most powerful and wealthy of all the Greek city-states, recently defeated by Sparta in the Peloponnesian war, briefly ruled by an imposed and vicious oligarchy of thirty tyrants, themselves supplanted by the most truly participatory democracy the planet has ever known. In classical Athens to be powerful and wealthy implied no contradiction with being cultured, compassionate, scrupulous and moral. Here it was that Europe first asked herself what her values were. Here for the first time it *mattered* to know what matters: to learn what was right, and to do it. Here the life of the mind and the life as lived in society were known to be inseparable, each expressing the other. Democracy was cherished and practised with a passion only recently rediscovered in Europe.

True, classical Athens was not, by today's post-socialist and post-feminist standards, unblemished. Of its 100,000 citizens, only 40,000 were franchised; women, slaves and resident aliens were relegated to democracy's sidelines. Athenians held wealth, status and physical excellence in high esteem. Yet they also valued the life of the mind, their philosophers forever enquiring into what it took to be most fully human, most fully developed in those intellectual and moral territories which demarcate the civilised from the barbarian.

The self-imposed mission of Socrates (c. 469–399 BC) was to see if he couldn't discover, for himself and with others, wherein lay the difference between right and wrong. His was a moral mission – to question anyone who professed to be wise. He sought simply to discover the nature of (in Greek) '*arete*': a word usually translated as 'virtue', but whose sense is perhaps better conveyed by 'excellence' or 'merit'. For Socrates held, with a fervour that was to cost him his life, that mankind's business on earth was to find out what was right, what was virtuous, and what was excellent. Socrates, like P. G. Wodehouse's Jeeves, satisfied himself that the place to look for answers was within the psychology of the individual. Socrates possessed in infuriating abundance the skill of bringing to the surface knowledge that was latent and nascent in the minds of all those who risked debate with him. His method, Socratic dialogue, was a process of guided introspection in which a chain of questions, each dependent on the previous answer, led his interlocutor (I nearly said 'victim') out of the maze of his own assumptions and ignorance towards insight. Socrates' further supposition (and it is a supposition we might not make today) was that once a person knew what was right and true his inevitable choice would always be to act virtuously on that knowledge.

Although Socrates himself left no written account of his own philosophy – he was that rare teacher, the man who wrote nothing but questioned everything – it is clear from the accounts of his principal trainee, Plato, that a coherent set of attitudes and beliefs underlay Socrates' career as a grain of sand in the oyster-bed of Athenian intellectual life.

In every human activity (Socrates believed) there are standards of attainment which, without always being able easily to define, we recognise as 'excellent'. We call excellence different things according to context: 'justice', 'honesty', 'skill', 'morality', 'courage' and so on. We do well to let a job be done by someone who possesses excellence in the particular field, and this applies alike to carpenters and doctors, thinkers and politicians. So it behoves the carpenter, the doctor or the politician to discover what constitutes excellence in his own sphere; to discover it, aspire to it, and train for it.

Socrates shared the universal suspicion that those in authority aren't always as meritorious as they think they are. Many of his recorded dialogues are with public figures, often wind-bags whom he pricks and empties of their unwarranted self-assurance like a surgeon incising an abscess. To the pupil thus deflated and made hungry for newer and better knowledge, the key question then becomes, "Can excellence be acquired by those apparently lacking it?". Socrates' dialogues show that, if nerve is kept and the process of awareness-raising questioning persisted in, not only *can* excellence be acquired, but the seeds of excellence can be found to be part of the innate constitution of all human beings.

The Sophists

In Greece at the time of Socrates, education had become a highly marketable commodity. Rapid changes in political and social structures had created a widespread need for higher education, especially in the areas of citizenship and leadership. A clique of itinerant teachers travelled from city to city offering instruction to anyone – usually the sons of rich and influential families – who wished it. These were the Sophists; and Socrates had many a bone to pick with them.

The Sophists' central principle, so far as they had one, was pragmatism. As a Sophist you taught what people most wanted; and what most people wanted to know was how to manage their personal affairs, how to regulate their households, and how, by speech and deed, to gain power and influence in public life. Train the offspring of the wealthy in the necessary skills, and you were well set up. If you were a Sophist, you expediently tailored your academic curriculum to the livery of your employer: you taught what suited. You would be more concerned to make your concept of 'virtue' resound well in the ears of the day's particular audience, but rather less concerned to tease out from it anything that risked being more fundamental, more universal, more radical and perhaps more subversive. So your definition of justice might be 'the laws of good law-givers'. Morality becomes a consensus phenomenon, not an ethical one. No matter! – who's to say what truth is? Truth, like cheap perfume, is a vapid luxury, quickly overpowered by the perspiration of the real world.

The skill the Sophists most loved to demonstrate and teach was oratory. In a civilisation where public speaking was the only mode of public influence, rhetoric – the ability to use language to evoke emotion, agreement and belief – conveyed immense power. A skilled orator could by rhetoric alone command the support of the democratic assembly. Small wonder, then, that the Sophists, most notable among them a certain Gorgias, claimed that oratory was 'the greatest and best of human concerns', and charged high fees for teaching a man how to induce conviction in his listeners. The Sophists' preferred educational vehicle was the lecture, their objective to gain applause rather than stimulate insight or self-awareness. Gorgias' descendants today would include Dale (*How To Win Friends And Influence People*) Carnegie, and a host of those running training seminars on Inter-Personal Skills for sales representatives and middle management. (And it has to be admitted that the list also includes those of us who today teach young doctors their consulting skills with models of four areas, five checkpoints, six phases or seven tasks!) [4–7]

More to the point, there are strong traits of Sophistry required to claim, as Trainers in General Practice have to claim to the committees that appoint them, the intention of teaching the Curriculum, the whole Curriculum, and nothing but the Curriculum. Herein, disguised as rigour, lurks another kind of academic pragmatism. 'Curriculum' hangs cosy but desiccating over education like high atmospheric pressure in a heatwave, first warming then scorching the sweltering land and resisting the essential encroachment of low pressure systems bringing invigorating rain.

To return to Socrates: because the Sophists' empirical view of excellence was so much at odds with his own urgent search for more durable and universally-based criteria, it is in his debates with the Sophists that we can most clearly discern the power of Socrates' dialectical style of teaching. Plato has recorded two very readable accounts of Socrates' encounters with Sophistry [8]. The conversation with Protagoras, the leading Sophist of the day, though brilliant, civilised and witty, concludes that they got themselves into a muddle because they had failed to agree at the outset on a definition of excellence acceptable to both. A second, shorter, dialogue which doesn't make the same error is that with Meno, a young aristocrat visiting Athens from Thessaly who had acquired a taste for philosophical combat from Gorgias himself. The *Meno*, which will take about half an hour to read, is a topic tutorial on what I have earlier called 'the locus of educational opportunity'; whether the fundamentals of self-development are innate, or dependent on an external authority. Socrates is able, by question and answer, to draw from the most entrenched student first the recognition of his own ignorance and need for knowledge, and secondly the realisation that he had possessed the knowledge he sought all along without realising it. 'In other words,' as Guthrie puts it in his Introduction to *Protagoras and Meno,*

> what is the secret of that peculiar quality which makes some men so much more proficient than others in the art of living according to the highest human capacities? Why do some men make a success of life and others a failure? Is it something we are born with or can it be acquired by taking thought, or instilled by the kind of instruction that a father gives his son or a master his pupil? [op. cit. p.9]

Picture (with a little dramatic licence for which I take responsibility) the scene.

Socrates' dialogue with Meno

It is 402 BC. Socrates, now in his late sixties and the target of official disapproval that will within three years have him executed for impiety and corrupting the minds of the young, sits on a wall outside the house of Simon the cobbler. Across the large open space of the Agora lie the great public buildings of Athens: the Senate, the city Archive, the Senate dining chamber. Seated most mornings on the wall outside the house of Simon the cobbler Socrates conducts his *'phrontisterion'* – his 'thinking-shop'. Around him is gathered his audience of young Athenians, too young still to be admitted to the civic business conducted in the Agora but already earmarked as the next generation of democrats. They are joined on this occasion by Meno – imperious, nobly-born, in Athens for a short time only, and intent upon gleaning whatever instruction he can from Socrates as quickly as possible. Taking for himself the 'hot seat', Meno weighs in with:

"Can you tell me Socrates – is virtue something that can be taught? Or does it come by practice? Or is it neither teaching nor practice that gives it to a man but natural aptitude?" [op. cit. p. 155]

A frisson of anticipation runs through the other students, for they have heard similar opening gambits before, and witnessed Meno's predecessors get their intellectual comeuppance.

"Well," begins Socrates guilelessly, "you chaps from Thessaly are used to experts like your friend Gorgias answering such questions with unerring confidence. I think you must have cornered the market in wisdom, for here in Athens all I can say is that, far from knowing whether virtue can be taught, I actually haven't the least idea what virtue *is*. So help me out; *you* define it for me."

Socrates' trap is sprung. Meno replies by giving examples of manly virtue, womanly virtue, the qualities of virtue in children, in old men, in slaves ... And would go on, did not Socrates press him to identify those general criteria of virtue which exist *independently* of the particular role or status of its possessor. Meno makes a couple of attempts which are painfully inadequate, amounting to little more than that virtue is the quality possessed by the virtuous. Socrates' promptings consist mainly of variations on, "I see; so by the same token you would say . . .", or "In that case, you would claim such and such; let's see whether that will stand up." Meno, who had thought the issue an easy one, is reduced to helpless protestation.

"Socrates," he cries, "you are like a sting-ray, paralysing anyone who touches it. Conversation with you is mind-blowing; you make my brain seize up!"

Which was of course Socrates' intention. He has made use of a process of dialectic known as 'Socratic *elenchus*' – a cyclical or reiterative questioning or testing of the pupil's stated position. Each successive tentative statement is measured against indisputable evidence and experience until any ignorance, fallacies and false assumptions become apparent. During the initial stages of *elenchus*, Socrates is at pains to treat Meno's vulnerable self-esteem with great sensitivity. Nevertheless, he has soon succeeded in evoking in Meno an awareness of a learning need, together with a desperate desire to have it satisfied. The sense of finding oneself on shifting sands, of discovering an unsuspected knowledge gap, of being compelled to doubt the validity of what had previously been taken for granted, is known to students of Socratic dialogue as '*aporia*'. *Aporia* translates as 'helplessness', 'confusion', 'doubt', 'being in a flap'. In a state of *aporia* the student recognises that his present state of knowledge simply won't do, but he doesn't yet know what is to supplant it. This conviction of ignorance is a necessary preliminary, clearing the ground for the beginning of wisdom. Meno's arrival at a state of *aporia* signals to Socrates that he is now maximally motivated to learn.

Now according to Plato, Socrates was often aware of a 'warning voice inside' which helped him keep his teaching on track. He called it his '*daimonion*' or 'spirit voice'; and although his critics, anxious to lay charges of heresy, interpreted this as a claim to be divinely guided, the *daimonion* seems to have been little more than Socrates' own preconscious mind alerting him just in time to the danger of going too far with his comments and losing empathy with his interlocutor. Meno follows his "sting-ray" jibe with the tetchy advice that Socrates shouldn't venture away from Athens, for anywhere else he would be arrested as a wizard. Meno's energy could obviously go either way – into angry dismissal or, more profitably, into curiosity and learning. The *daimonion* has spotted this moment of crisis.

So now Socrates changes tack. He abandons his previous adversarial approach. Instead he quite genuinely aligns himself with Meno's discomfiture and offers him a way forward which both can pursue without loss of face.

"It isn't that, knowing the answers myself, I willfully perplex other people", Socrates reassures Meno. "The truth is rather that I infect them also with the perplexity I feel myself. So with virtue now. I don't know what it is. You *thought* you did, but now it seems *you* don't either. Nevertheless I'm ready to carry out, together with you, a joint inquiry."

Meno gratefully agrees, although he wonders, since neither of them knows what they are looking for, how they are to recognise it if they find it. Socrates is familiar with this apparent paradox. "This is a trick argument, this claim that a man cannot try to discover either what he knows or what he does not know; that he wouldn't bother looking for what he does know, and in the other case doesn't know what he ought to be seeking."

Meno is intrigued. "Why's it a trick?" he asks. "What's wrong with it?"

Socrates is said to have paused, for this is a solemn moment. Anticipating Jung's idea of the 'collective unconscious mind' by two millenia, he replies (and I paraphrase):

"Some part of human nature – call it the 'soul' if you like, or 'collective wisdom' if you prefer – is immortal. It dies and is reborn with each generation, but is never finally extinguished. It has learned everything of importance that *needs* to be learned. The world doesn't change in its essentials, so when a man has recalled a single piece of knowledge there is no reason why he should not find out all the rest, if he doesn't grow weary of the search. For seeking and learning are in fact nothing but recollection."

"Prove it," says Meno. So Socrates does: not by a further display of verbal dexterity, but with a practical demonstration. "Call one of your slaves over. Does he understand the geometry of squares and square roots? Does he know how to construct a square double the area of a given square? Of course not, you say. I say he does, though he thinks he doesn't. Be sure to listen carefully, and see whether I'm telling him the answers, or whether through my questioning he's simply being reminded of principles he already knows."

And Socrates draws squares in the sand at the slave-boy's feet. The slave first reckons that "obviously" a square of twice the original area has a side twice as long. When this is seen not to work, he guesses that the square root of 2 (for this is the concept being pursued) is one and a half. Wrong again, he discovers. The slave doesn't know where to turn next. He has been touched by the sting-ray. Meno of course knows how he feels. The geometry experiment is an exact analogy for his own discussion with Socrates on where to search for excellence. Yet he will allow that the slave's impasse has done him no harm, merely serving to render him receptive to the further promptings of his common sense in response to Socrates' questioning.

Socrates starts his 'square' diagram afresh, this time subdividing it into four quarters, whose diagonals the well-questioned slave can clearly see form the desired square of side $\sqrt{2}$. Quod erat demonstrandum [9]. Meno acknowledges that although Socrates asked the right questions, the supposedly ignorant slave himself supplied the necessary acumen and intuition. Socrates nevertheless counsels caution. "At the moment your slave's grasp of his new knowledge is rather precarious. But if similar questions are put to him repeatedly, he'll soon have as good an understanding of geometry as anybody. What's more, not having learned it parrot-fashion from someone else, he'll be able to expound on the subject to others with real authority."

Socrates' educational objective has not been an arcane and ultimately sterile argument on the immortality of the soul. Instead he has used the vivid analogy with the slave to liberate Meno from the stranglehold of his own assumptions and show that the search for fresh knowledge is a fruitful one. He and Meno are now free, intellectually and (more important) attitudinally, to continue. After reaching the block, and gaining confidence that there is a way around it, they are ready for the next phase of tuition. Socrates, whose own mother had been a midwife, calls this 'theatetus', or 'mental midwifery' – bringing into the light of day ideas which were latent in the other's mind. To use his own metaphor, theatetus is "assisting the delivery of ideas with which the other was pregnant".

The dialogue with Meno progresses to wonder, as we must as well, how all this fits in with training in specific skills such as shoe-making, doctoring and flute-playing, and (by implication) government. The group is joined by a prominent politician, Anytus, who is a spokesman for Philistine views of the "What you don't know won't hurt you" kind. Anytus seems to feel that Meno, in his quest for excellence, would do far better to latch onto any decent working Athenian gentleman, and stay away from smart-alecs like Socrates, agonising over epistemology and educational theory. "Find yourself a thoroughly admirable man, a statesman like Themistocles or Pericles, or Thucydides the historian. Stick with him, and you might learn something!" "A shame, though", Socrates gently chides him, "that the sons of all three were thick as two short planks; and the fathers could teach nothing of excellence even to their own children."

Anytus flounces off. Three years later he is to be one of those prosecuting Socrates on capital charges of over-effective teaching.

Oh what a powerful teacher is story-telling. As Anytus stomps away, and Meno is left wistfully contemplating what with a little effort he might become, and Socrates' tutorial group disperse to their homes and into history, we might well wonder whether anything much has changed in twenty-five centuries. But if the dilemmas are eternal, so are the answers. Nowadays, as teachers struggle to foster curiosity and probity in pupils beset with massive informational work-loads, the legacy of Socrates was never more precious.

The legacy of Socrates

In 1972 a book, *The Future General Practitioner – Learning and Teaching*, was published which laid the foundations for what has become the highly successful enterprise of Vocational Training for General Practice in Great Britain [10]. Written by the then lions of General Practice education, it established a secure basis not only for the core curriculum of General Practice but also the educational methodology of one-to-one and small-group teaching. It espoused the orthodox model of how to teach, known as the Educational Paradigm (Figure 1.1).

From a job description are inferred general goals, which can be itemised as specific and testable objectives. Teaching strategies are employed to teach these objectives, and assessment methods used to define the content and method of subsequent teaching.

In their section on Teaching Styles, the authors of *The Future General Practitioner* list 'Socratic' as one style, alongside 'authoritarian', 'heuristic' (finding out for oneself), and 'counselling' [op. cit. p. 218 ff]. A 'Socratic' style is rightly presented as 'teaching by question and answer. The teacher always asks and the learner always answers. It is essential that each answer be the trigger for the next question.' The Socratic style, the authors claim, 'seems to be an inherent ability and is not easily learnt.'

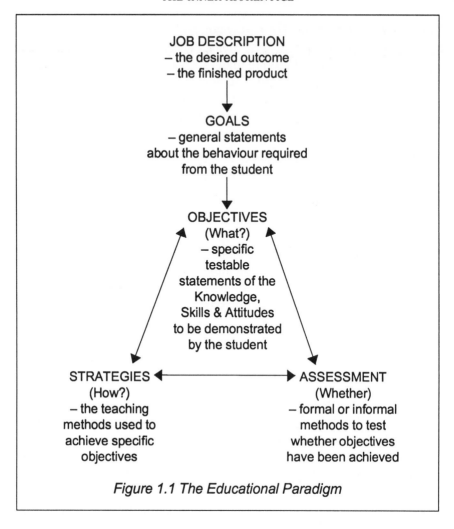

Figure 1.1 The Educational Paradigm

They warn against a drift into authoritarianism, and offer an example that to my mind does Socrates considerably less than justice.

I hope, however, that on the strength of what I have so far presented the reader will already have a sense that Socrates' educational legacy is potentially far more complex and valuable than this. Perhaps, after our eavesdropping on the dialogue with Meno, a number of ideas and questions are already forming in the mind, together with a curiosity to see whether we can identify and to some degree replicate Socrates' undoubted effectiveness as an educator. The elaboration of these ideas and questions into concepts, strategies and methods appropriate to contemporary post-graduate education is one part of the agenda for the remainder of this book.

The dynastic impulse to 'show'

Socrates clearly had so fervent a passion for teaching that, when convicted for corrupting the minds of the young, he preferred death by hemlock to enforced retirement from his chosen career. During his speech in mitigation, when banishment was suggested as an alternative punishment, he said, "I know very well that wherever I go young people will listen to my conversation, just as they do here. Someone may say, 'Surely, Socrates, you can spend the rest of your life quietly minding your own business.' How can I make you understand? To let no day pass without discussing goodness and all the other matters I debate with myself and with others – this is the very best thing a man can do. Life without this sort of examination is not worth living."

What can motivate a man to such an extremity of idealism? Contemporary sources tell of Chaerephon, his childhood friend, returning breathless from Delphi early in Socrates' philosophical career having asked the Oracle there whether anyone in the whole world was wiser than Socrates, and having received the unusually explicit answer "No". We learn how Socrates, flattered yet perturbed by the prophecy, embarked on a series of interviews with the reputed sages and experts of the day – public figures, teachers, poets, playwrights and craftsmen – finding each on close examination to be self-deluding. He described this quest as "a sort of pilgrimage", leading inexorably to his oft-quoted conclusion that "the only thing than can be known for sure is that nothing can be known for sure." But is this a slogan worth dying for? It may well be, as Socrates himself maintained, that the citizens of a democratic society require from their leaders expertise in clear thinking comparable with the manual skill required of their carpenters; and that he had a knack of being able to cut through self-deception in those professing to be wise. But Socrates had no wish merely to be acknowledged 'right'. Rather than trade insults with his intellectual opponents, Socrates instead spent his life in a series of personal involvements with self-selected students, attempting to foster self-critical habits of thought which would allow them to create excellence for themselves. This seems to speak of motivation at a deeper level than mere intellectual assertiveness or vainglory.

The teacher's traditional account of his vocation runs something like this: "There is such a thing as human fulfilment, and such a virtue as assisting the young to attain their personal approximations to it." Without detracting from this altruism, I think there is more to it than that – certainly in the case of Socrates, who was not known for his self-effacement, and probably in our own. It seems that the life of the mind is subject to a kind of 'dynastic impulse', a mental equivalent of the biological urge to reproduce children in one's own lineage. We long to have a new generation value ways of thinking that we ourselves have come to value; to have someone else see what we ourselves have seen and found delight in. The rising generation affords more opportunities for us to meet such aspirations than do our own immediate peers. Our contemporaries, whose ideas are already formed and as precious to them as ours are to us, are more likely to respond to a challenge with contradiction, irritation and rejection. The young, on the other hand, hold out the prospect of curiosity, appreciation, even gratitude and respect, as well as a rejuvenating scepticism. Conceited though the acknowledgement of such factors may make us appear, I believe they are important motivations for most teachers. Like all psychological forces, they can be channelled either for good or ill: it is our professional responsibility to ensure the former.

I remember the jolt with which, in 1973, I first saw this dynastic impulse acknowledged on a theatre stage. Peter Shaffer's stunning play *Equus* narrates the encounter between Martin Dysart, a child psychiatrist, and Alan Strang, a boy from a 'good' home who has blinded six horses [11]. In this excerpt Dysart has begun to understand Alan's passion and rather to envy it. His own wife is a brisk no-nonsense Scottish dentist with no enthusiasms, no passion. He confides to a woman friend:

> Occasionally I still trail a faint scent of my enthusiasm across her path. I pass her a picture of the sacred acrobats of Crete leaping through the horns of running bulls – and she'll say: 'Och, Martin, what an *absurred* thing to be doing!' . . . Mentally, she's always in some drizzly kirk of her own inheriting: and I'm in some Doric temple – clouds tearing through pillars – eagles bearing prophecies out of the sky . . . I wish there was one person in my life I could show. One instinctive, absolutely unbrisk person I could take to Greece, and stand in front of certain shrines and sacred streams and say 'Look! Life is only comprehensible through a thousand local Gods . . . I'd say to them – 'Worship as many as you can see – and more will appear!' . . . If I had a son, I bet you he'd come out exactly like his mother. Utterly worshipless.

Ground rules of Socratic dialogue

From Plato's accounts of his mentor's dialectic style, we can see that Socrates adhered closely to certain pre-conditions and procedural principles to ensure effective *elenchus* and keep the dialogue on track.

Agreement on agenda: The interlocutors should agree at the outset on the purpose of their discussion, e.g. to discover whether excellence is teachable, or to establish the hall-marks of good public speaking.

Agreement on definitions: Most of Socrates' enquiries were into abstract qualities like excellence, skill or piety, which can mean different things to different people. Clarification of this potential misunderstanding is a prerequisite of fruitful discussion (and sometimes *all* that is required, though the clarification can take a long time). Socrates always insists on a general definition, rather than a succession of examples. For instance, in considering a definition of skill, particular cases of skilled behaviour will not do: what is required is agreement on what all examples of skilfulness have in common. By this means, the interlocutor's all-important value systems become accessible for discussion.

Questions, not statements: The aim of Socratic dialectic is not merely that clarity should emerge, but that the interlocutor should feel the pride of ownership of that clarity. Given this aim, and Socrates' working assumption that everyone has access at some level to the necessary insights, it follows that the emphasis in discussion needs to be kept on the interlocutor's opinions as they emerge in succession and are progressively refined. Questioning is the effective means of doing this, as a tennis coach might throw a series of easy balls over the net in order for a pupil to practise ground strokes.

Answers beget questions: As an antidote to the inhibitory effect of asking too many closed questions, we are often told, "If you only ask questions, all you get is answers." The traditional remedy is the open-ended question, such as, "Would you like to tell me about . . . ?" The danger here is of an overly discursive and probably judiciously censored reply.

The Socratic alternative would be the aphorism:

> *Let each answer beg the next question.*

If the teacher takes up each question at the point where the previous answer has left off, the exploratory tip of the student's inquisitiveness is kept on the advance, like the pseudopodium of an amoeba sensing nearby food. This need not be done oppressively. There are many ways, direct and indirect, of asking a question. But the teacher's contribution in a Socratic discussion is confined, so far as possible, to questioning and clarifying the pupil's moment-by-moment train of thought rather than imposing his own.

Commitment to one's answers: It is important that the interlocutor should believe in the answers he makes, and that questions should be asked in a way that makes this safe. Otherwise the enquiry remains academic, so that when the stage of awareness of a deficiency of knowledge (aporia) is reached, the student remains uninvolved and disinterested in the resolution.

Balancing challenge and support: There is great vulnerability involved in having one's knowledge and beliefs scrutinised. Risk-taking of this nature needs to be respected and sensitively balanced with a sense of support. To coin a phrase, we learn best in safe insecurity. It is apparent from the irritation that his interlocutors frequently show, and from the controversy that attended him, that Socrates despite his 'warning voice inside' often fell short of the ideal balance.

A new Socratic paradigm

Reference has already been made to the 3-stage Educational Paradigm, the teaching cycle of Objectives, Strategies and Assessment (see page 19.) In Socrates' teaching method we can discern an alternative model for the emergence of insight, applicable at least on the brief time-scale of a single tutorial encounter and probably over a more extended period of learning as well. Socrates' educational paradigm started from an agreed topic, inferred those concepts needing an agreed definition, and then embarked on a 3-stage process of *elenchus* (testing by question and answer), *aporia* (awareness of a learning need), and *theatetus* (allowing intrinsic wisdom to emerge) (Figure 1.2).

Figure 1.3 presents this more simply, and in a way that may make clearer its potential application in contemporary vocational education.

The encounter takes place within a relationship which both participants have defined as educational. One takes responsibility for leading discussion, and the other willingly adopts the role of learner (though this role need not prevent his views from ultimately prevailing). Systematic and thorough self-disclosure by both parties leads to clarification of the relevant assumptions and value-judgements that each is making. Careful Socratic questioning then enables each to discern the knowledge gaps or attitudinal barriers preventing progress. The nub of the issue is perceived particularly acutely by the pupil, who feels a compelling need to learn in order to preserve self-confidence or self-respect. Further skilled questioning by the teacher calls forth from the pupil exactly those innate resources of intellect, intuition or perception needed to restore a sense of self-esteem.

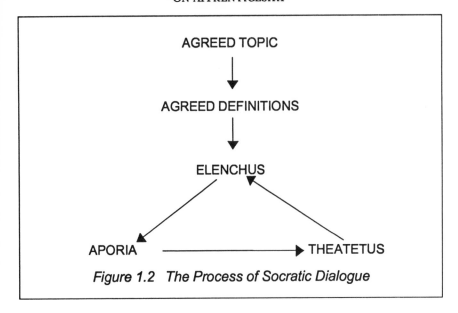

Figure 1.2   The Process of Socratic Dialogue

'The Teacher Within'

Plato on several occasions mentions Socrates' *daimonion* – the still small voice inside him which would warn him when he was talking his way into trouble. Socrates himself sometimes refers to it as if it had some supernatural origin, but his tongue is in his cheek. I think in fact Socrates was using his interlocutor's minimal cues – facial expressions, body language, speech patterns – as a form of feedback. He would pursue some point that seemed to him intellectually relevant, but at the same time constantly monitor the other's behavioural responses to confirm receptivity and check for agreement. When he registered signs of disagreement or a weakening of rapport he would immediately deal with these more pressing concerns before continuing. In other words, his intuition kept his intellect on track. Although it may initially seem daunting to seek to cultivate such an intuition ourselves, a few moments spent recalling the poorer teachers of our own school-days will confirm its importance.

Pre-resident knowledge

Maintaining as I am the need for a rediscovery by today's teachers of the key elements of Socratic teaching style, I anticipate several problems. Just how far is it fair to push the correspondence between the purely philosophical issues Socrates addressed and the vast array of facts, concepts and values that entrants to professions must master nowadays? Whatever it was that Socrates meant by '*arete*' – virtue, excellence, quality

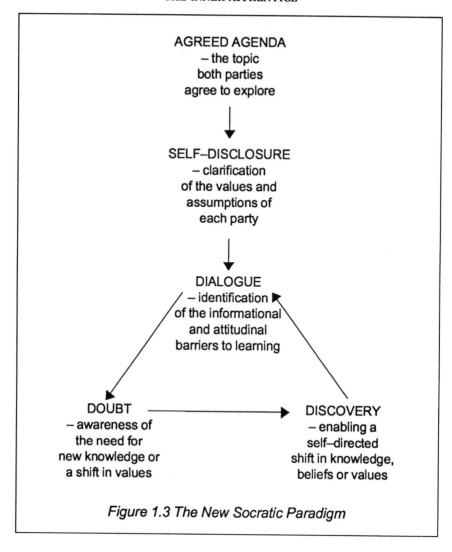

Figure 1.3 The New Socratic Paradigm

— and whether or not it should prove to be learnable — surely Vocational Training cannot and should not be over-simplified to such a naive abstraction? Education Socrates-style is a process akin to open-cast mining, with awareness-raising questions clearing away the topsoil and impedimenta layer by misguided layer until the valuable insight-bearing ore is revealed. But just what *is* this insight or pre-resident knowledge we allegedly all can possess? The ability to fall in love, or to tell kindness from cruelty, or to grasp the axioms of simple geometry — if these are what is meant, we might allow them. But knowledge of the date of Magna Carta or the dose of penicillin, certainly not. And what of attitudes and values, such as compassion or inquisitiveness — are these 'virtues' to which all may give birth if attended by a Socratic midwife?

And even as we begin to bridle, the legacy of Socrates is at work, asking us the questions which carry us to the heart of our pre-suppositions, unsettling us, and denying us peace of mind until we understand things better.

An analogy with a modern computer may help keep our questions on track. A computer is a system for manipulating information. User-specific information (Random Access Memory, RAM) is brought into interaction with pre-resident non-alterable information (Read-Only Memory, ROM), according to processes some of which are pre-installed in the computer's Disc-Operating System (DOS) and others of which are programmes chosen and loaded by the user. There are however two further types of computer memory of interest to teachers. Programmable Read-Only Memory (PROM) is installed by the user, not by the manufacturer, but cannot be altered after initial installation. It resembles the 'tabula rasa' of the new-born baby, the blank sheet of memory on which early experience leaves its indelible imprint. In computer parlance, DOS and ROM would be 'nature', while RAM and PROM are 'nurture'. The second even more interesting is EPROM, Erasable Programmable Read-Only Memory. EPROM is also 'taught' to the computer by the user, and remains constant during ordinary use. But it can be 'un-learned' and re-programmed if the user so wishes, by a sequence of instructions carried out separately from ordinary daily use. Once incorporated, EPROM functions as permanent memory until the next time it is re-programmed. EPROM is 'permanent for the time being', and in the analogy is the domain of the teacher.

If we overlook the anachronism, Socrates is asking us to discriminate more carefully between RAM, ROM, PROM and EPROM. Perhaps the content of the human read-only memory is greater than we thought. Perhaps some of the human characteristics we believed immutable and beyond the reach of teachers are after all programmable, and erasably programmable at that. Perhaps it's just that our usual teaching methods, working mainly with short-term Random Access Memory, are inappropriate ways of influencing medium-term and long-term memory stores. And perhaps, most exciting of all, better ways await our discovery.

The personal touch

Early on in this chapter I feared for the safety of what, for want of a better phrase, I called 'the personal touch' in vocational education. Socrates had the personal touch; in fact, he insisted on it. He refused any other way.

Socrates himself, for all that he was clearly fond of the sound of his own voice and enjoyed renown, left no written accounts of his philosophy. Most of what we know of him comes from the memoirs of his friends, notably Plato, who recorded his mentor's conversations, often years after they took place, in 'Dialogues' of unlikely fluency. Here is Socrates talking to Phaedrus on the subject of book-learning:

> It shows great folly to suppose that one can transmit or acquire clear and certain knowledge of an art through the medium of writing. (It's like painting. Portraits may look like living people,) but if you ask them a question they maintain a solemn silence. The same holds true of written words; you might suppose that they understand what they are saying, but if you ask them what they mean by anything they simply return the same answer over and over again. Besides, once a thing is committed to writing it circulates equally among those who understand the subject and those who have no business with it; a writing cannot distinguish between suitable and unsuitable readers. [12]

Socrates was convinced that only the collaborative format of here-and-now one-to-one cut-and-thrust dialectic could lead a particular pupil to the particular insight which on that particular occasion he was ready for. Curiosity expressed at a distance is for peeping Toms; wisdom acquired at a distance is parrot-learning; for two people who are serious about self-enhancement, the encounter is everything. Have you ever read a book with as much passion as you have argued over a late-night coffee?

I referred earlier to the two ascendant models of education as processes either of quest or revelation, which differ in their 'locus of educational opportunity': in the one the locus of opportunity resides within the pupil, and in the other it is with the teacher. From Socrates we learn of a third option. In the Socratic encounter the locus of opportunity is in the *relationship* between the two. Here we have the origin of a third model – 'education as *Apprenticeship*'. The impetus for learning by apprenticeship comes from neither individual but rather from the relationship between them: from its ground rules; from its interplay of psychodynamics; from its willingness to question all assumptions and to shun collusion; and above all from its value system that establishes as its first priority a pupil's longing for completeness.

'Follow-through'

History is silent as to what, if any, was the lasting impact on his interlocutors of their encounters with Socrates. We know that the course of his principal apprentice Plato's life was changed as his awe of Socrates mellowed into admiration and friendship. Though his own philosophy developed considerably after Socrates' execution, Plato is nowhere more compelling than when narrating the events and encounters of Socrates' life and championing his reputation. In 386 BC, embittered by his friend's fate, Plato founded his Academy in Athens, the world's first University. Its aim (to breed a new and honest type of politician) and methods (the study of logic, ethics and Socratic dialectic) are documented in the world's first text-book of education, *The Republic* [13].

But we don't know the intellectual fate of Meno, of Protagoras, of Gorgias, of Phaedrus and the others. Being cross-examined with the penetrating thoroughness of Socrates can't always have been fun. Were their lives nevertheless gratefully enlightened, or did they slink off, chastened men, clutching the remnants of their shredded self-esteem and vowing never again to risk the discomfiture of change? Probably neither extreme was the case. Probably some blind spots were illuminated, some fresh lines of thought opened up. The point is, the outcome of Socratic dialectic was unpredictable. Socrates could not know whether his one-off encounters produced lasting and valuable psychological and intellectual growth. His implied assumption that they did itself demands Socratic challenge. There is evidence to the contrary in the list of those inter-locutors who subsequently vilified him and, in the case of Anytus whom we met briefly while talking to Meno, actively petitioned his death.

In a word, what Socrates lacked was 'follow-through'. However effective his process of dialectic may have been on the short time-scale of a single tutorial encounter, he seems not to have had a corresponding facility for ensuring that the processes he started were carried through into lasting change in the medium and long term. We should not blame him for this. But we should learn from it. A facility for dialectic needs to be matched by skill in managing the trajectory of apprenticeship. Learning in its early stages is synonymous with vulnerability. It needs the protection and reassurance of a supportive emotional environment. The pupil's insecur-ity is, in the course of time and under favourable circumstances, capable of evolving into discovery, challenge, self-discovery and self-motivation. Then a different form of facilitation is called for, one which can aid in the melding of each fragment of learning into a greater process. Skill in structuring and pacing the trajectory of apprenticeship – follow-through – is the necessary complement to Socrates' gifts as a tutor.

THE RELATIONSHIP OF TUTELAGE

There are clearly many areas of complex human attainment calling for education and training of a greater order of magnitude than a single Socratic encounter, or even a series of them. A student seeking proficiency and excellence in art, in craftsmanship, in an academic discipline, in the professions or in sport must expect, and should demand, a carefully thought out process of sustained and enduring maturation. Different cultures and different historical periods have all solved the problem of educational follow-through in much the same way – apprenticeship. In apprenticeship, the Socratic principle of personal engagement with a skilled mentor becomes extended in time over a period of months or years. Within this longer time-scale fresh dynamics begin to operate. The Socratic paradigm remains an appropriate model for individual pieces of learning. But the success or otherwise of uniting the components of theory, practice and values into an overall trajectory comes to depend more on the evolving relationship between teacher and pupil than on any one tutorial encounter.

This 'relationship of tutelage' between master and apprentice is the necessary extension of, and framework for, the effective one-to-one teaching exemplified by Socrates. Lucky the teacher who can combine Socratic facility with a grasp and command of the greater relationship, and lucky the pupil of such a one. Let us take encouragement from a few instances of successful tutelage, and learn from them. As evidence that the deep structure of apprenticeship is universal, I'll take three diverse examples: from the Europe of the Middle Ages; from the Hollywood film industry; and from sport.

The medieval craft guilds

In Europe from the 10th century onwards, as the requirements of a civilised life grew to exceed the resources of any single one of its local communities, the institutions of commercial intercourse were born. Artisans and craftsmen produced commodities – cloth, metalwork, pottery, wine, works of fine art – which would allow an individual town to barter its way out of temporary adversity after a ruined harvest or civil disruption. Troops of merchants travelled the Continent, compelled by the threat of attack by armed marauders to gather into companies, like wagon trains, for mutual protection. Safety lay in solidarity.

Mankind creates an institution out of every instinct. Out of nervousness were created the craft guilds of medieval Europe. The craftsmen were nervous of the fickleness of their customers; consumers were suspicious of the arcane knowledge of the craftsmen; both needed the protection of a system they could trust to regulate the emergent professionalism of the new crafts. Throughout Italy, France, Germany, the Low Countries and England the same social forces produced during the 11th and 12th centuries the same solution – the craft guilds. The medieval craft guild was a corporation enjoying the monopoly of practising a particular art, trade or profession in accordance with regulations sanctioned by public authority. And while it must be admitted that craft guilds could be charged with protectionism, conspiracy against the laity and stifling healthy competition between practitioners, they did nevertheless afford some benefits to the populace. Minimum acceptable standards could be defined and a measure of reliability and accountability introduced. Not least, however, and of interest to us now, was the emergence of a system of training by apprenticeship, controlling entry into crafts whose potential market was not limitless and which were therefore concerned only to take in new members skilled enough to maintain standards of proficiency.

At the top of the craft hierarchy were the craftmasters, their numbers restricted by the local market, independent entrepreneurs owning their own premises, tools and materials, and the output of their workshops. At the bottom were the apprentices, working for little more than their keep and tutelage in the craft, and the chance of eventual admission, on production of an acceptable 'masterpiece', to the rank of master. In between masters and apprentices were the journeymen, who had served their apprenticeships but had not yet fulfilled all the financial, social and civic criteria required of a master.

Let Marx, if he will, develop from this state of affairs a critique of class exploitation and political oppression. Such iniquities notwithstanding, there is still much to be learned from the educational processes underlying the progress from apprentice to journeyman and master. In particular, because of the long periods of time involved, training in the medieval craft guilds allowed what we might think of as the natural history of apprenticeship to become discernible. Apprenticeship in medieval Europe can teach us about what I have referred to as 'trajectory'.

The most perceptive description I have come across of the dynamics involved in apprenticeship, in which the parallels with contemporary Vocational Training can be clearly seen, comes from a surprising source – an account of the spiritual values of modern art by an American art historian and scholar, Dr Roger Lipsey [14]. The following passage from *An Art Of Our Own* is from a section headed 'Joys of the Apprentice, Sorrows of the Journeyman' [op. cit. pp. 180–184].

The mystique of tradition is complex. It is made up in part of a sense of immersion in an enduring enterprise to which one comes as a neophyte, a learner and beggar. . . It recognizes the difficulty of certain traditional ideas, which may require a lifetime to understand with the whole of one's being. . . Participation in a strong tradition is experienced as inviting, even as a necessity for one's life, but also as forbidding. Because there are standards, there is the risk of failure. . . The aspirant goes forward nonetheless, and this is the beginning of a modest sort of heroism.

Apprentice, journeyman, master – these are the stages of initiation into craft traditions and, by extension, into any tradition that demands effort over long periods of time. When the aspirant has recognized the tradition to which he or she *must* belong and has obtained provisional acceptance as a student, the ecstasy of apprenticeship begins. The central experience is guided learning under the tutelage of an impressive teacher. A hitherto unknown world of ideas and methods is freely opened to the apprentice. The tuition and menial service associated with apprenticeship . . . are nothing in comparison with the opportunities for learning. The abuse meted out to the apprentice for errors made and ideas misunderstood is nothing in comparison with the limitless joy of being given another chance. Learning itself is redefined as an assimilation not only of external methods and intellectual concepts but also of attitudes, customs, history, sensibility. The apprentice enters into a tradition as if into a great house with innumerable rooms, each to be visited and memorized, each containing a test of his or her substance and adding to it.

All this occurs under the eyes of the mentor. To be a child in such a house and of such a father or mother is a great thing, entailing only a child's limited responsibility. Needless to say, the apprentice's admiration for the mentor is boundless. Every word, every gesture has meaning. The poor mentor cannot even tie a shoelace unobserved . . .

The apprentice in time becomes the journeyman. Scarcely less joyful in its earlier stages, the journeyman's life is one of provisional companionship with the master and marked by the assumption of limited teaching duties, not so much to teach as to learn in greater depth. The journeyman knows many of the techniques of the craft, although there is still much to learn; . . . (he or she) is well on the way toward *becoming* the craft and need not always look outside for a sense of direction. The journeyman recognizes with increasing clarity that the tradition exists only *in and through people*, not in the abstract, and that it must be carried on through a fragile human medium; hence a dawning sense of responsibility, well before the journeyman is capable of full responsibility . . .

This duality in the end becomes a burden: the journeyman is neither child nor adult, neither joyously tied to the mentor nor wholly free. A dark time ensues. Admiration for the mentor is increasingly accompanied by unspoken recognition of his or her shortcomings, perhaps not in the craft itself but in other respects – and perhaps even in the craft because no one, finally, is all things.

The relation between journeyman and mentor is by now old and well established; it easily survives these small depredations. More serious is the journeyman's uneasy sense of being over-shadowed by the mentor, as if some maturation, only guessed, is impossible at close quarters. . . The mentor, seeing more than he or she lets on, leaves this miserable situation intact for a long time. It is the final fire. No amount of compassion can relieve it. Furthermore, the mentor himself experiences a subtle change of heart. He cannot help but see that his teaching has failed in many respects; the journeyman is acceptable, perhaps even shows mastery on occasion, but more often seems living proof that the teaching was clumsy and unworthy of his own teacher's example.

At this stage of the drama, the mentor traditionally invites the journeyman to produce a ritual object known as the "masterpiece" . . . to demonstrate to senior members of a craft guild that the journeyman deserves a place among them. . . Judgement and acceptance of this object are not left to the journeyman's mentor alone, for he or she is not expected to be objective. For the occasion, a number of masters of the craft gather around. If all goes well, the masters induct the journeyman into the craft as a mature worker in whom they deem the full authority of the tradition to be intact.

Now a master, and prepared in turn to be a mentor, the former journeyman may discover what it was that remained out of reach. The final level of mastery cannot be conferred by others.

If he succeeds in making that discovery, the tradition will continue to grow; if he fails to do so or forgets that it is needed, the tradition will begin, perhaps unnoticeably, to wither. For the goal of the drama just enacted is to bring individuals to the point where they not only sustain a tradition but add to it.

I don't suppose that life as an apprentice goldsmith amidst the squalor and drudgery of the Middle Ages was in reality anything as ecstatic and inspirational as Lipsey, dwelling on its more visionary aspects, portrays in his account. Nevertheless there is something about the apprentice's pilgrimage from ordeal to initiation and apotheosis that brings a lump to the throat. Empathically we imagine ourselves experiencing, and perhaps in due course bestowing, a similarly fecund and committed opportunity. Lipsey's 'ecstasy of apprenticeship' is more than just a phrase: it's a phrase that resonates. A note of rhapsody is there within us all for the sounding.

For some that note may be a call to action; for others a requiem for lost possibilities. We sense intuitively that within a relationship of tutelage are buried the seeds of everything we might be and the husks of everything we might have been; and the knowledge moves us.

The universality of this wistfulness – the fact that we respond at all – is the point. Apprenticeship medieval-style is still alive. It must be – it makes good movie box-office!

'The Karate Kid'

"Only the 'Old One' could teach him the secrets of the Masters", runs the logline to Jerry Weintraub's unashamedly poignant film *The Karate Kid* (Columbia Pictures, 1984). Danny, a fatherless teenager from America's East coast, is uprooted to California, where he becomes the target of bullying by the Cobras, a vindictive gang of karate students with a charlatan teacher. By chance Danny's handyman, Mr Miyagi, is a true Master of the martial art. Danny comes to believe that he too might acquire Miyagi's skill, and with this vision comes the hope of survival. The old man initially plays hard to get, which only strengthens Danny's resolve. The training is at first more gruelling and less heroic than Danny had envisaged. It seems to consist merely of endless chores – painting fences, polishing floors, cleaning cars. In fact, unbeknownst to all except Miyagi, Danny is acquiring proficiency in the muscular coordination and mental concentration required of a true karate student. Realisation that his training has been skilfully master-minded only dawns when in the film's climax Danny defeats the Cobras' leader in combat and gets the girl. Hackneyed and sentimental, yes – and millions-of-dollars-worth true. Younger viewers empathise with Danny, older ones with Miyagi, but the film's success indicates that the relationship of tutelage is recognised as being one not only of great value but also one which contemporary material values place in jeopardy. When we watch the film, we're rooting not only for Danny but also for the method – the apprenticeship – to win through.

If we look beneath *The Karate Kid*'s all-too-easily-dismissed surface structure we can discern some of the deeper features which make apprenticeship at the same time desirable and risky, a source both of potential satisfaction and potential embarrassment. The apprentice is naive, an underdog, potentially a victim of those more experienced, needing skills he doesn't at first know exist if he is to survive in his chosen world. The teacher sees in the apprentice a means of immortalising accomplishments which might otherwise die with him. (In the sequel

Karate Kid II we learn that Miyagi's 'dynastic impulse to show' comes from his need to atone for a long-past episode of immaturity and inadequacy.) Their relationship is not a mere liaison of convenience but one of mutual advantage at emotional and motivational levels. The apprentice's final coming-of-age is a significant transition for teacher as well as student.

Athletes and coaches

As I write, World Cup football dominates the television. So far there has been more energy and passion on the managers' bench than on the field of play, as they try by shout, gesture and telepathy to influence their teams. Soon it will be Wimbledon. Between games the camera will linger on the faces of the players' coaches, unnaturally impassive as they struggle to contain the involvement they are feeling with their protégés' fortunes.

David Hemery won the gold medal in the 400 metres hurdles at the 1968 Olympic Games. Since his own athletic prowess peaked, he has devoted himself to studying how athletes in various sports at all levels can be helped to fulfil their sporting potential. His book *The Pursuit of Sporting Excellence* describes the conclusions he reached after interviewing 63 top performers in 22 sports [15].

As might be expected, natural physical endowments, family upbringing, and attributes such as courage, competitiveness, concentration and self-discipline are all important elements. Not least, however, is the relationship between athlete and coach. 89% of Hemery's sample set store by their experience of coaching. Interestingly, several top athletes, including Ian Botham, Greg Chappell, Arnold Palmer, Lester Piggott, Steve Davis, Chris Evert Lloyd and Sebastian Coe, had been coached by their fathers. 40% of his sample rated the coach–athlete relationship as intensely significant. It seems there is a range of coaching styles that can be equally effective. Many however seem to have in common a balance between authority (an uncompromising insistence on discipline and dedication) and a personal concern for the athlete's overall well-being off the field. This unfeigned caring, says Hemery, "is the binding ingredient which makes the authoritarian approach on the field understandable and therefore accepted by the athlete."

Hemery identifies a number of aspects of coaching where matching between coach and athlete is needed if the relationship is to succeed. (Perhaps surprisingly, technical accomplishment by the coach is not a *sine qua non*.) First, their aims and priorities must coincide: each must understand and accept the other's vision of the goals of their work together, and these must be realistic, not falsely idealised. Secondly, there must be mutual respect for each other's skills, and confidence in each other's abilities; without this, faith and trust diminish. Thirdly, each must pledge the necessary commitment of time and effort. It is easy for an athlete to underestimate the time commitment made by the coach, particularly in the early stages of training. The coach's input evolves during the course of their relationship as with experience the athlete increasingly becomes 'self-coaching'. A skilled coach can achieve an imperceptible transition from a coach-centred to an athlete-centred style of training.

The word that keeps cropping up, however, is *motivation*. The good coach is the effective motivator. It is not necessarily the case that the coach motivates the athlete by his own infectious enthusiasm; cheer-leaders don't always make good coaches. Rather, the good coach is one in whose presence the athlete's own motivations are brought to peak intensity. The coach somehow manages to convey to the athlete a sense of the greatness which is within his grasp, and more importantly, a vision of another and another level, previously unimagined, to which he may yet aspire. Together, coach and athlete explore the same trajectory as Mr Miyagi and the Karate Kid, master and apprentice.

EDUCATION AS APPRENTICESHIP

A later chapter will develop some specific techniques from the self-evident similarities between sports coaching and vocational education. For the present it is enough to establish that the psychodynamics of apprenticeship, from Socrates to Hollywood, are well appreciated, if not always well understood. Earlier in this chapter I distinguished between two current deep structures of education, Revelation and Quest. If we could combine the best of the Socratic process of teaching by awareness-raising with the transformational power of a long-term relationship of tutelage, we should have, I believe, the ingredients of a third option – 'education as Apprenticeship'.

In the 'Revelation' view of education, the driving force behind learning – the locus of opportunity – was seen to be *external* to the student. The teacher is all-responsible. In the 'Quest' model, the locus of opportunity is *within* the learner; the teacher is pure facilitator. A view of education as 'Apprenticeship', however, places the locus of opportunity firmly *in the relationship between teacher and pupil*. If we are concerned to improve the outcome of higher professional training, our attention must focus on enhancing the effectiveness of the interplay between the two parties as their relationship evolves moment by moment, day by day, and month by month.

It has been said that "When the Pupil is ready, the Master appears". Neither the readiness of the Pupil nor the appearance of the Master is by itself sufficient; both are necessary, and each creates the other. In apprenticeship, both in the Socratic short-term and in its long-term trajectory, the teacher's constant aim is to mobilise usable curiosity in the pupil. At the same time, it is by correctly perceiving the pupil's ever-changing state of readiness that the teacher keeps his interventions on track. The teacher is forever divining by whatever means he can – from intuition to formal assessment techniques – what the pupil is on the point of needing to learn. He then translates that readiness into the opening up of a succession of spaces into which he knows the pupil can expand. The pupil is kept, like a toddler learning to walk, constantly toppling forwards into outstretched arms. Without the risk of the topple he would not move; without the outstretched arms he wouldn't even try; without the unbalancing there would be no exhilaration. Learning occurs in safe insecurity.

It is strange that our system of Vocational Training for General Practice, which is so clearly and securely cast in the apprenticeship mould, remains rather coy about it. One of Britain's major contributions to General Practice as an academic discipline, stemming from the work of Michael Balint and his associates, has been the recognition that the unconscious forces operating between doctor and patient are no less important than the superficialities of their encounters. We seem rather reluctant to extend this insight to encompass the complexities of the relationship between a Trainer and Trainee. It seems to be not quite nice. We cheerfully, even proudly, maintain that in becoming a mature practitioner a Trainee has first to acknowledge, then to express, and finally to discipline the wilful forces of his own unconscious life – instincts, fears and conflicts as well as the more acceptable qualities of creativity, emotionality and intuition. But we prefer this insight to be bestowed as it were at arm's length, handled cautiously lest it drop off and mark us with the stain of vulnerability.

Certainly I am aware as I review this chapter that in advocating apprenticeship as an appropriate model for Vocational Training, I touch upon psychodynamics which we may feel nervous of conceding. The emotional trajectory of a traineeship is identical to a normal parent–child relationship, with issues of bonding, sibling rivalry, Oedipus and Electra complexes, adolescent rebellion and so on, culminating in separation and the empty nest. Many potentially dangerous issues are present, even if they are not openly addressed: power, dominance and control; sexuality; the negotiation of boundaries and personal space. Visible or invisible, these are ever-present forces in every relationship of tutelage. It is tempting to distance ourselves from them, and to take flight into structured curriculum and assessment methods. But we thereby play down the personal touch and renege on the central truth that the primary vehicle of learning *is* that very relationship. A new neurosis seems poised to become endemic amongst Trainers – 'influence anxiety'. Its symptoms are: a willingness to accept payment for instructing the young; a dread of being thought manipulative; curriculophilia; pathological self-effacement and feelings of unworthiness; and a morbid fear of admiration.

Perhaps the hardest pill for teachers to swallow is the notion that we might after all be heroes. Suggest that we quite intentionally aspire to the heroic role of apprentice-master, and everything British inside us goes off at once. We shrink from so conceited an idea: modesty forbids, and all that. But what's wrong with heroes? For every person who could use a hero (and who could not?), someone else has to *be* one. Better even a reluctant hero or heroine for a role model than a curriculum check-list. Socrates, the medieval master-craftsman, Mr Miyagi, Seb Coe's dad – all have managed to wear with grace the mantle of heroism. Heroism is but a seasonal garment; to don it need be no hypocrisy, no vanity; and to shed it once outgrown is an act of strength, not of weakness. Perhaps, masochists that we are, we have stared so long at our navels that we see only frailty and unworthiness there. Dared we but lift our heads and return our pupils' gaze, might we not with honour see reflected in their eyes a brow bedecked with a laurel crown?

Part II
The Icarus Factor

Ah, but a man's reach should exceed his grasp,
Or what's a heaven for?

Robert Browning

Chapter 2
The story of Daedalus and Icarus

TRAINS, NETS AND WILL-O'-THE-WISPS

Teachers, like railway engines, run on a track with two rails. One – call it *faith* – is the gut feeling that there is such a thing as human completeness, that is, making the most of oneself. The other – call it *mission* – is the urge to be working alongside individual students, assisting them towards their own personal versions of that possibility. To be sure, synonyms for 'completeness' can sound disconcertingly like left-over argot from the Age of Aquarius: 'self-actualization', 'the fulfilment of human potential'. And to be sure, the pure energy of vocation is often sapped as inevitable compromises are made to routine, prejudice and sheer human frailty. Nevertheless, a teacher need only reflect upon the opportunities of his own life-span or fondly recall the achievements of certain students to know that growth, both personal and professional, is no mirage. The twin rails of faith and mission must and can run parallel. If either should buckle or deviate, the spiritual wounds sustained by all on board are no small disaster.

We have seen, as we traced its pedigree through a succession of historical and cultural guises, how apprenticeship is an appropriate model for the educational environment of today's professionals in training. At this stage much detail still remains to be worked out. In principle, though, apprenticeship combines faith in human perfectibility with the mission and methodology to advance it. Earlier I have warned against relying too heavily either on an imposed curriculum or on laissez-faire self-discovery. However, we cannot postpone indefinitely identifying precisely what it is we wish the experience of apprenticeship to bring about in vocational trainees. The '*how?*' must have its '*what?*'.

In the field of Vocational Training for General Practice, *The Future General Practitioner* supplied the first systematic account of the attributes of the 'successful' graduate [1]. True to the principles of the traditional Educational Paradigm, it starts with a job description inferred from observing what good doctors do (or would do in an idealised reality!).

The general practitioner is a doctor who provides personal, primary and continuing medical care to individuals and families . . . He accepts the responsibility for making an initial decision on every problem his patient may present to him, consulting with specialists when he thinks it appropriate to do so . . . (He) will work in a team and delegate when necessary . . . His diagnoses will be composed in physical, psychological and social terms. He will intervene educationally, preventively and therapeutically to promote his patient's health. [Op. cit., p. 1]

From this job description are derived eleven broad goals describing the objectively measurable 'patterns of behaviour a trainee should be able to demonstrate on completing vocational training'. These are comprehensive and laudable. They include:

- making diagnoses expressed in physical, psychological and social terms;
- demonstrating how recognition of patients' individuality modifies the clinical process;
- demonstrating reliable decision-making;
- demonstrating the special use of time in general practice;
- demonstrating an understanding of the effects of family relationships and social characteristics on illness;
- making use of a wide range of therapeutic interventions;
- demonstrating skill in effective practice management;
- continuing to meet his own educational needs;
- understanding the methods of medical research; and
- auditing his own work willingly and critically.

With snowballing enthusiasm, the authors of *The Future General Practitioner* and their academic successors have further rubricised these goals into the familiar triad of 'Knowledge', 'Skills' and 'Attitudes'. These they have expanded into five 'broad divisions of educational objectives':

- recall of factual knowledge;
- performance of manual skills;
- employment of knowledge and skills;
- demonstration of interpersonal skills; and
- demonstration of self-understanding.

These last two are an acknowledgement of the difficulty in assessing attitudes other than by noting their effects on observable behaviour. A further classification of objectives groups them into five 'areas':

- Health and diseases;
- Human development;

- Human behaviour;
- Medicine and society; and
- The practice.

Finally, Vocational Training abounds in versions of a core curriculum, consisting mainly of home-spun check-lists and confidence rating scales with several hundred individual items, each of which the Trainee is invited to cover [2]. There is by now a significant body of literature developing these principles into a comprehensive and well-articulated discipline.

Phew! I refresh the reader's memory of all this not to decry it, but to pay tribute to the very great investment of time, thought and resources that has gone into providing a sound academic base and an effective infra-structure for Vocational Training in Great Britain today.

Ungrateful and seditious of me, therefore, to ask, "Does it all work as well as it might?" Perhaps, but I'm going to. Most Course Organisers and Trainers design their courses and tutorials more or less explicitly towards meeting defined objectives in each of the three cardinal areas, Knowl-edge, Skills and Attitudes. However, it seems to me that we teachers feel a lot more at home with the knowledge and skills part, and distinctly on edge when it comes to attitudes, particularly those concerned with the personal and professional values of our Trainees. For General Practice Trainees, the three years of their Vocational Training, and especially their year's traineeship in practice, is a period when the pattern of their long-term professional behaviour is established. That Trainees change and mature during their training is obvious; that the direction and magnitude of that professional and personal maturation owes much to our conscious educational strategies is less apparent. Fulfilment and excellence should be the goals, and deserve to be the destiny, of anyone embarking on a Vocational Training. Apprenticeship – the relationship of tutelage – seems to be mankind's best shot so far at devising a process for bestowing them. The trouble is, 'fulfilment' appears to be a will-o'-the-wisp; and despite our chasing it with a net made of objectives and check-lists, 'excellence' tantalisingly evades capture, no matter how fine the mesh. We shall have to sneak up on it with rather more circumspection.

DAEDALUS AND ICARUS

Eric Berne, the Transactional Analysis man, first documented the rules of the universal game of "Ain't It Awful" [3]. In it two people who consider themselves the victims of misfortune restore their self-esteem and console each other by alternately describing an escalating series of hard luck stories. Trainers, while not professional players of "Ain't It Awful", are keen amateurs. They have devised a version, best played in small groups of four or less, called "Ain't Training A Struggle". As they compare notes with their peers, one will masochistically boast how difficult, how insensitive, how incompetent, how unresponsive, how lazy is the Trainee now in post. "That's nothing," say the others, "mine doesn't even, couldn't even, wouldn't even . . ." Before long a group gloom is established. Someone will mention silk purses and sows' ears. Another will say, "At least we tried", and all will nod; and someone else will start talking about better formative assessment tools, and all will nod more vigorously and promise themselves another bash at the video, the check-lists and the rating scales.

Quite often, however, (and this is more likely in larger groups), the mood will suddenly flip. "Mind you," someone will say in a lighter tone, "they're not all like that. You remember so-and-so, whom we all adored, who never prescribed antibiotics for colds, who said my tutorials were really helpful, who did a project on 'heart-sink patients', and who walked on water?" The chorus agrees. "Teaching's really fun when you get someone who doesn't seem to need teaching." A heady mix of nostalgia and optimism takes over, and the game changes to "Ain't Training A Breeze". Baskers in reflected glory that we all are, the lucky Trainer will bow the head in false modesty and murmur, "I like to think, you know, shucks, in some small way, maybe I helped, or rather, was able to facilitate . . ." And again, all will nod more vigorously and promise themselves another bash at the video, the check-lists and the rating scales.

It does seem to be the case that the same educational process can for some young doctors provide a springboard to rewarding and committed professional lives, while for others it is at best a life-belt and at worst a strait-jacket. There seem on one hand to be 'high-flyers' who take off and soar, and on the other pedestrians, who lurch through their training, never get off the ground, and who may sooner or later fall by the wayside.

The question has to be asked: "Why?" What are the differences between the high-achievers and the average or under-achievers? What is 'the difference that makes the difference'? Can we – or even should we – do anything about it? Is it all in the genes and the pre-school years? (If it is, what are we doing agonising over teaching methods and taking money for it?) Are the two extremes the way they are because of or in spite of anything their Trainers did? How can we discover and release whatever potential is latent within each Trainee? What forms of teaching, guidance or experience are most likely to help our Trainees make the most of their individual talents and interests? In what ways might our teaching be different in order to help make the difference that makes the difference?

These questions formed the starting point for a programme of study for which I was lucky enough in 1988 to be awarded the inaugural Fellow-ship of the Association of Course Organisers. This book is the result of a search for some answers. Its conclusions can be summarised thus:

> *People are intrinsically self-educating,*
> *as long as the right information is provided*
> *in the right way at the right time.*

But I am getting ahead of myself. First I want to retell an old story. Stories and metaphors are safe but powerful ways of opening us up to the possibility of things being different. Stories resonate with and restimulate the curiosity we had as children. They raise spiritual and moral agenda for us in a non-threatening way. 'Meta-phor' means a carrying beyond; stories prepare us to be carried from what we already know into the realm of what we might discover. A verse of Emily Dickinson's includes the lines:

The Possible's slow fuse is lit
By the Imagination.

Many cultures ask the really important questions and teach the really important lessons in the language of gods and heroes, allegories and myths. In Robert Graves' compendium *The Greek Myths* is recounted the archetype of the Trainer–Trainee relationship [4].

The story so far: Daedalus, a famous Athenian craftsman, took a succession of apprentices. One of them, his nephew Talos, so far exceeded his master in skill that Daedalus out of jealousy murdered him. He fled to the island of Crete, where he enjoyed great renown as a carver of wooden dolls. Daedalus became the world's first known sex therapist. One of his successful projects was a behavioural technique for mating King's Minos' wife Pasiphaë with a white bull belonging to Poseidon the sea-god, a coupling which resulted in the legendary Minotaur. The king, peeved, imprisoned Daedalus and his son Icarus in a labyrinth, from which they sought to escape. Now read on.

Daedalus made a pair of wings for himself, and another for Icarus, the quill feathers of which were threaded together, but the smaller ones held in place with wax. Having tied on Icarus' pair for him, he said with tears in his eyes: "My son, be warned! Neither soar too high, lest the sun melt the wax; nor swoop too low, lest the feathers be wetted by the sea." Then he slipped his arms into his own pair of wings and they flew off. "Follow me closely," he cried, "do not set your own course!"

As they sped away, . . . the fisherman, shepherds and ploughmen who gazed upward mistook them for gods.

(Soon) Icarus disobeyed his father's instructions and began soaring towards the sun, rejoiced by the lift of his great sweeping wings. Presently, when Daedalus looked over his shoulder, he could no longer see Icarus; but scattered feathers floating on the waves below. The heat of the sun had melted the wax, and Icarus had fallen into the sea and drowned. Daedalus circled round until the corpse rose to the surface, and then carried it to the nearby island now called Icaria, where he buried it. [Op. cit. vol. 1, pp. 312-3]

The tale of Icarus and his fate is a surprisingly powerful and fruitful analogy for us now. Some of its correspondences are profound, others humorous; all are instructive.

The reason for Daedalus' murder of Talos is interesting. According to Graves, twelve-year-old Talos happened upon the jawbone of a serpent, and found he could use the serrated teeth to cut a stick. He copied the jaw in iron and thereby invented the saw. This and others of his inventions, including the potter's wheel and the compasses, secured for Talos a great reputation in Athens; hence Daedalus' jealousy. In a gesture reminiscent of the 'urge to show' described by the psychiatrist Dysart in the passage from *Equus* quoted earlier, Daedalus led Talos to the summit of Athene's temple on the Acropolis – and toppled him to his death! Here we have an extreme example of some of the psychological forces at work in the relationship of tutelage. The 'normal' Oedipal pattern, in which son longs to murder father, is reversed. The journeyman's increasing mastery of his craft serves to underline the fallibility of the master's own skills, a tension which (as Lipsey described) could have been better resolved had Talos been allowed to survive and undergo the ordeal of 'graduation by submission of masterpiece'.

When we come to the actual flight of Daedalus and Icarus its aptness as a metaphor for Vocational Training becomes even more apparent. The 'father–son' transference relationship between master and apprentice has in the myth become literally true, but not quite legitimate: Icarus' mother Naucrate had been a slave in King Minos' household. The labyrinth, which Daedalus himself had originally designed, is a self-constructed rut from which escape has become urgent if our heroes are to break free to new possibilities.

The idea of salvation through flight seems to have come from Daedalus. In a rather didactic, Trainer-centred and 'spoon-feeding' way he constructed not only his own wings but also those of Icarus. There was no initial formative assessment, no cooperative clarification of the youngster's wishes. In the design of the wings, the more solid construction of the main quills showed good coverage of the core curriculum, but tragically insufficient attention was paid to the higher-order objective of securing the smaller feathers.

Daedalus cautions against excessive soaring or swooping, and forbids Icarus to follow his own autonomous course. By this well-intentioned advice he unwittingly sets the trap which awaits every mediocre teacher and his pupils, namely the assumption that "there is only one way – my way!" The flight will succeed if, and only if, curiosity and exhilaration are forsworn and the trajectory is flat and undemanding. By his warning, Daedalus shows that he has recognised Icarus' secret wish to out-fly his father. Because his strategy has failed to take account of this normal adolescent reaction, and because of the inflexibility of their flight plan, Daedalus' presentiment of disaster becomes self-fulfilling. Icarus, we presume, was not suicidal. He merely supposed that the risk he knowingly took had been foreseen by him whose business it was to foresee it. Learning, as I have suggested, requires conditions of 'safe insecurity'. In this case the safety proved illusory and the insecurity unrecognised; with disastrous results.

Presently – 'presently', for Heaven's sake!; what use is 'presently'? – presently Daedalus looks over his shoulder and realises what has happened. We can imagine the scene later in the Coroner's Court on Icaria.

Coroner:	Exactly how did your son come to fall into the sea?
Daedalus:	I can only assume –
Coroner:	I'm afraid we must deal in facts. Was the sun hot that day?
Daedalus:	No hotter than usual.
Coroner:	And the wax of its usual quality?
Daedalus:	Yes, I always use the same brand.

Coroner: And your own flight was uneventful?

Daedalus: Yes, yes! *(sobbing)* I blame myself. If only I had checked behind me more often, or let him fly ahead of me. Then I'd have seen what was happening.

Coroner: There there, don't distress yourself. You did everything you could. This is a case of the foolhardiness of youth, nothing more. I shall enter a verdict of death by misadventure.

But if I were the Chairman of a Trainer Selection Committee, I should ask some awkward questions when Daedalus next came up for re-approval. And if I were the Chief of Police on Icaria, and the Criminal Records Office in Athens told me what had happened years earlier to Talos, I should, as they say, make further enquiries.

The beauty of stories is that however they finish, they never end. A story tossed into the mind is like a stone leaving ripples that pattern the surface of a pond long after the stone has sunk. Metaphors and myths engage us at levels deeper than facts do; a well-timed metaphor is immortal, and has a greater power to create new and lasting wisdom than any logic or research. A story inspires in proportion to its endlessness. Indeed, it is by the fact that a good story won't go away that we can tell it has a message for us.

I first used the myth of Daedalus and Icarus as a metaphor for Vocational Training in an article in the British journal *Postgraduate Education for General Practice* [5]. Shortly after it appeared, I had a letter from Dr David Haslam, a highly-esteemed General Practitioner and writer, whose mind was rippling from the splash of that particular pebble.

"There is", he wrote, "a fundamental flaw in the whole Icarus legend. Supposedly the higher Icarus flew, the nearer the sun, and the quicker the wax melted. But – as you go higher, it actually gets colder, even though you are nearer the sun. So the wings should have functioned more efficiently at a higher altitude. In fact, those who fly high are more prone to burn-out than to melting. The heat is generated from within."

"The heat is generated from within." Is Haslam merely playing with words? If so, my riposte would be that Daedalus wouldn't have known where the fatal warmth came from, as he hadn't been looking. Besides, in mythological times the sun was only just out of arm's reach, not millions of miles away; so obviously, the higher the warmer. But this is not the right level of response; Haslam's is not an adversarial comment. As the physicist Niels Bohr once observed, "The opposite of a deep truth is another deep truth." Haslam, by his new twist, enables the story to reveal yet another layer of relevance. Or rather the story, encountering Haslam, crystallises for him another layer of his *own* insight; namely, that people, however enthused they may be by good example, also possess an internal energy which can either uplift or destroy, according to circumstance.

Images and stories have the power to re-associate parts of our knowledge which were in danger of being dissociated. An excellent book on this psychotherapeutic potential of metaphor, *Mutative Metaphors in Psychotherapy* [6], takes as its keynote a line by Gaston Bachelard, a French philosopher and scientist who died in 1962. The line, which has echoed and re-echoed since I first read it, is timely:

But the image has touched the depths
before it stirs the surface. [7]

Chapter 3
The hallmarks of excellence

Icarus the heat-seeking, the heat-generating, the heat-sensitive: what *is* it, this 'heat', this energy at the same time attractive and dangerous, intrinsic yet seemingly out of reach? What *are* those smouldering qualities in Trainees which, well-tended, can waft them safely onwards and upwards but which, injudiciously fanned, can end in spontaneous combustion? It is time to move on from myth and metaphor and for this enquiry to take a more practical turn.

That for which 'heat' has been a metaphor in preceding pages is the pupil's potential for excellence. In the last chapter we noted how medical teachers have no difficulty in recognising that excellence, whatever *that* means, is something displayed by different Trainees to differing degrees. Being good latter-day pupils of Socrates, we must press the question, "What *is* 'excellence'?" And we'll begin, as most of Socrates' pupils would have done, by seeing if we can identify the hallmarks of excellence in the context (but not the exclusive context) of Vocational Training.

So like Meno I asked myself, "What *is* 'excellence' in the context of Vocational Training, and is it teachable?" I decided to start by finding out what other medical teachers meant by excellence, and also by seeing what might be learned from other professions where excellence of some kind was at a premium. Much work on professional excellence has been done in the commercial world of business and industry, and it was here I looked first to see whether some of its lessons would prove transferable to the medical setting.

COMMERCIAL EXCELLENCE

Browse amongst the shelves of any airport bookstall and you would think, to look at the non-fiction titles, that the high-flying traveller had only two obsessions – 'executive success' and how to attain it; and 'executive stress' and how to conquer it. (Smart guys, these airport bookstall managers, peddling simultaneously both the cocaine and the Valium of corporation life.) If you're a middle manager or a fledgling entrepreneur with fantasies of becoming another Lee Iacocca, or a Victor Kiam, or a Michael Edwardes, all you have to do, it seems, is study their commercial hagiologies. Buy the book, learn the lesson, model the hero, transform the company, become the tycoon: such is the implied promise. Here's a typical advertising puff:

> Executive success. You don't have to go to Japan for it, nor can you achieve it in one minute. . . Today's crisis-ridden manager needs more than a quick fix to meet the challenge of this New Age of constant change. Strategic planning alone can't do it. Neither can corporate culture-building. *Creating Excellence* proposes a rational yet visionary blend of both approaches for a winning, strategy-driven culture that can take you and your company into the twenty-first century with the confidence that gets results. Based on a programme of six essential leadership skills – vision, sensitivity, insight, versatility, focus and patience – this step-by-step blueprint for organisational excellence shows the New Age Executive exactly how to:
> Make the most of your firm's capabilities;
> Motivate your people to peak performance;
> Respond positively to change from within and without;
> Develop long-term goals and see them through;
> And turn crisis into opportunity. [1]

Yes. Well. Possibly. Or if that looks like fool's gold, how about *Leadership and the One Minute Manager – Increasing Effectiveness through Situational Leadership*? Or perhaps *Peak Performers – The New Heroes in Business*: 'a must-read for all those who prize increased performance and productivity'? As I leafed through these titles it became increasingly hard to resist their optimism. I felt like the man at the convention of whirling dervishes who only does the waltz. What I had taken to be a healthy scepticism on my part started to seem very Puritan and small-minded. Cynicism began to evaporate, and I found myself reacting more with curiosity than with disdain. Maybe the Californian jargon and the jet-set razzmatazz, garish and ersatz though it might at first appear to jaundiced British sensibilities, might nonetheless have some lessons for us. I read a little more of *Creating Excellence*. The authors seemed to feel about the traditional business curriculum much the same as I did about the orthodox paradigm of medical education.

Most business schools (they wrote) teach six fundamental managerial skills that supposedly insure (*sic*) success in today's business world:
- set goals and establish policies and procedures;
- organise, motivate and control people;
- analyze situations and formulate strategic and operating plans;
- respond to change through new strategies and reorganizations;
- implement change by issuing new policies and procedures;
- produce respectable growth, profitability, and return on investment.

While these may have worked in the past, declining American productivity and competitiveness prove they no longer suffice. To achieve corporate excellence in the dynamic future, managers must learn to transcend the past with what we call the New Age skills:
- *Creative Insight* (asking the right questions)
- *Sensitivity* (being able to bind a team with shared motivation to achieve high goals)
- *Vision* (having a clear imagination of how things might be)
- *Versatility* (anticipating change and being comfortable with novelty)
- *Focus* (orchestrating resources towards a desired goal)
- *Patience* (having a sense of the long term as well as the short).
  [Op. cit. pp. 30–34. My paraphrases in brackets.]

If these are the hallmarks of excellence in today's commercial world, I have to confess I like them. Leaving aside for the moment the issue of how far a person can be trained in these general qualities, as descriptions of attributes desirable in doctors as well as managers I would have no quarrel with any of them. Intrigued, I read further; and was impressed by *Peak Performers: The New Heroes in Business,* by Charles Garfield [2]. Garfield was a world-class weight-lifter who turned to clinical psychology after working on the highly motivated Apollo space programme that put an American on the moon to please President Kennedy. He knows about excellence, having made a study of high achievers in a variety of fields, mainly commercial, and he introduces his study thus:

There is a kind of everyday hero whom many of us admire: the man or woman who possesses the ability to achieve impressive and satisfying results, not just once or twice but repeatedly, consistently . . . (Such peak performers) may not be so different after all. Now we can see that the differences between peak performers and their less productive co-workers are much smaller than people think – that extraordinary achievers are ordinary people who have found ways to make a major impact . . .

(Peak performers are) people who translate mission into results. They are always willing to evolve and grow, to learn from the work as well as complete it, to be "better than I was before." . . . The peak performer's ability to function is neither a singular talent nor even a collection of skills, but an overall *pattern* of attributes. Possessing these attributes, a peak performer will very likely:
- be motivated towards results by a personal mission;
- possess the twin capacities of self-management and team mastery;
- have the ability to correct course and manage change.

(For peak achievers) the starting point is an internal decision to excel. Until that decision is made, nothing much will happen. Thus we arrive at the key question: How do we get ourselves and others to commit, to make that internal decision to excel, and to develop ourselves in the process? One peak performer speaks for most others when he replies, "I got jump-started by watching others, by learning from the people I most admire." The peak performers say repeatedly that stories of our most productive people provide them not only with strategies but also with values – values as leverage points for triggering that impulse to excel. Why do human beings care so much about some things that they will concentrate every resource on them? For answers, look to their values.
   [Op. cit. pp. 15–18]

IN SEARCH OF EXCELLENCE AMONG TRAINEE GPs

One of my own intellectual heroes, though I never met him, was the psychologist Abraham Maslow. Maslow was one of those who inaugurated what has become known as the 'humanistic' school of psychology, which locates the main-spring of all human attainment and well-being firmly within the capacities for self-expression and self-fulfilment which are the inheritance of every human being. In his immensely valuable book *Motivation and Personality* Maslow gives an account of the study which energised the whole of his subsequent career [3]. Whereas most of the patriarchs of psychology from Freud onwards had taken as their raw material the human mind distressed, and had therefore a greater understanding of psychopathology than of mental health, Maslow tackled the subject from the opposite end. He investigated a cohort of people who by general acceptance were at the peak of mental and emotional fitness, and sought to identify those parameters which defined them as such. He was thus able to describe a set of qualities, hierarchically arranged and about which more will be said later, that were the hallmarks of individuals who had been able to fulfil their intrinsic potential to the fullest degree.

Feeling that a similar approach might serve my present purposes, I constructed a questionnaire and sent it out to as many of the Course Organisers of Britain's Vocational Training Schemes as I could locate. The two central questions I posed were:

(1) Are there any Trainees, on your Scheme at present or who have finished within the last year, whom by your own criteria you would describe as 'outstanding'? Please list, in as many particulars as you can identify, what it is that makes them outstanding.

(2) If you can think of any Trainees who have *not* fulfilled their potential as you perceived it, could you indicate what it is that you regret?

101 Course Organisers replied; and presently I'll report on their collective wisdom as to what it is that makes a 'good' Trainee good, and a 'bad' one bad. First, however, I need to set their replies in context. It was immediately apparent that, by asking what I naively thought were straightforward questions, I had poked a stick into a hornets' nest.

Most of my respondents could easily discriminate and describe those qualities which, to them, made the difference between outstanding and disappointing Trainees. Some, however, were suspicious of the exercise. It seemed to smack of elitism; although high and low achievers clearly do exist, to discriminate between them, even anonymously, was felt by some to be an act of disloyalty to those judged weaker. Although it might be nice if everybody could be 'excellent', not everybody can be; and there was a fear that if too much attention was paid to the high-flyers, the others might lose out.

"I am afraid that I cannot in truth approve of your scheme," wrote one Course Organiser. "I feel that we should concentrate our energies to the task of helping young doctors in our 'own patch' to become good, safe GPs, in order that the service to the public will be gradually improved. This is more important than looking for and fostering 'outstanding' Trainees. One may be able to change people's attitudes and develop enthusiasm, but I do not think it is possible to change a person's basic ability. . . The profession in my experience has been bedevilled by elitism in the not too distant past, and anything that fosters that kind of development should be discouraged."

Another reply: "I have been carrying your letter about with me for days discussing it with my colleagues and family. I find it impossible to answer the questions you ask. We seem to produce an encyclopaedic list of all our carefully selected Trainees, each one excellent in some aspect of personality, and the more we think about it the more their excellence seems to consist of how much we like them. . . In some ways it is like asking who do you love most: to which the only answer is 'I love all sorts of people in all sorts of ways'."

It seemed to a third "that we should be aiming at a reasonably all-round GP in our Training Schemes, and that identification of those doctors with excellent qualifications is not likely to raise the standard of the other 90% who are struggling to be turned out as safe, competent GPs. . . It is difficult to see Trainees fulfilling any sort of potential while they are still in the moulding process on the training year."

Nevertheless the comments of other Course Organisers encouraged me to continue. 101, the number of my respondents, was also the number of Disney's dalmatians, which are either white dogs with spots of black or black dogs with patches of white. The Course Organisers, similarly dappled, seemed in their teaching roles to divide into two camps. Most were basically hopeful but with spots of educational gloom that they could use some help with. Others sadly sounded chronically pessimistic, with just enough moments of cheer to keep them going. The *cris de coeur* of this latter group confirmed that there is indeed an important area of professional training for which the traditional approach is insufficient. "Very interesting project," one respondent wrote in a postscript to his reply. "It may rewrite the rule book. I do hope so!" Somebody else wondered, "Does Vocational Training achieve anything more than the passage of time?" "I don't know if the Trainee year has made a scrap of difference," echoed another. "The years of hospital training seem to squeeze out all academic interest." "Underachievement in Vocational Training has been the norm." "Oh the problems we have at the lower end of the scale, teaching people who have little knowledge and less aptitude!" And my favourite – "I regret corporal punishment's not available."

THE HALLMARKS OF MEDICAL EXCELLENCE

When I reviewed my 101 questionnaire replies, it was fairly easy to 'cluster' the Course Organisers' opinions of desirable qualities under 14 headings. These are summarised in Figure 3.1, and I'll explain and expand on each in turn. The percentage figure after each trait indicates the proportion of Course Organisers who identified it as a significant

RESPONSE TO NOVELTY (41%)
'CARITAS' (40%)
CLINICAL COMPETENCE (37%)
SELF–AWARENESS (35%)
'GROUP–ABILITY' (34%)
PERSONAL QUALITIES (30%)
EDUCABILITY (29%)
MOTIVATION (28%)
BALANCE (20%)
INDUSTRY (19%)
COMMUNICATION SKILLS (16%)
MISSION (15%)
CRITICAL ABILITY (7%)
DIVERSITY (7%)

(Percentages indicate number of Course Organisers
identifying the trait, $n = 101$)

*Figure 3.1 The 14 hallmarks of excellence in
Trainee General Practitioners*

factor in their own appraisals. Where possible, I quote the actual words used by the respondents. As you read each item, try keeping a part of your mind separate to ask, "Does conventional teaching reliably inculcate these qualities; and if not, why not?"

Response to novelty (41%)

The single most valued quality in Trainees is a positive and welcoming response to all the new ideas and working methods that Vocational Training exposes them to. Their teachers love to introduce them to fresh ways of thinking, but need to be met half way by a reciprocal curiosity from the Trainee. Typical comments included: "excited by new ideas, by challenge and change", "innovative and original", someone with "intellectual curiosity", who "grasps new concepts easily", who perceives "ignorance is a challenge, not a threat", and who is "intrigued by, yet sceptical of, new ideas".

On the other hand Course Organisers are frustrated by a Trainee who is "not prepared to widen horizons" and "unable to tolerate uncertainty", who has "rigid and unbending attitudes", and who, having been "brutalized by hospital medicine" is "unable to shift from a 'hospital' style of medicine".

'Caritas' (40%)

Of equal importance are those qualities of genuine caring for patients summed up in the Latin word *'caritas'*. The motto of The Royal College of General Practitioners, *'Cum Scientia Caritas'*, emphasises the complementary roles in family medicine of clinical competence and compassion. Outstanding Trainees care. They are "sensitive", "good listeners", "empathetic and understanding"; they are "approachable" and "patient-centred", have a "real interest in people as individuals", and "can relate to all social classes".

Clinical competence (37%)

It was reassuring to confirm that the importance of clinical skill had not been overlooked in the educational navel-gazing my enquiry prompted. Almost without exception, those Course Organisers who mentioned it at all put clinical competence at the top of their list of desirable attributes. They like a Trainee who not only "has sound reliable clinical skills", but who also "keeps her knowledge base up to date" and "keeps abreast of current literature".

Self-awareness (35%)

Course Organisers set a premium on Trainees' ability to recognise their own strengths and weaknesses. 'Self-awareness' includes not only self-assessment of clinical and educational needs, but also familiarity with one's own psychological landscape, and insight into one's own motives, needs and feelings. Some described this quality as "personal integrity" and mentioned being "able to ask for help". But many respondents seemed to find it easier to speak in terms of its opposite: "unable or unwilling to reveal his or her own humanity and vulnerability", having to "extract personal needs from the doctor–patient relationship" and "neglecting patients he dislikes". They had evidently found some Trainees "defensive", "lost in the 'doctor' image" and "unable to handle an 'open' approach". They were worried by "lack of confidence", "poor self-esteem", and by Trainees who might be "unable to confide in their Course Organiser".

Interestingly, a few sexist opinions were discernible. Male doctors were thought "more likely to be defensive and resistant to change than female"; some apparently have "highly defensive personalities, and can be highly disruptive, nit-picking, and very difficult to change." Women, on the other hand, were thought "more likely to drop out of Vocational Training".

'Group–ability' (34%)

My questionnaire had been sent to Course Organisers, who do most of their formal teaching in a small group setting; unlike Trainers, whose primary vehicle is the one-to-one tutorial. Not surprisingly, therefore, a valued attribute in Trainees is the ability to use a small group effectively. Small-group work is widely, and probably correctly, credited with the power to bring about a significant degree of psychological maturation, through exposure to peer opinion and the special dynamics which operate in groups. The 'parent–child' transference of the relationship between individual Trainers and Trainees is, in psychodynamic terms, a more primitive stage in emotional evolution. Thus the ability to feel comfortable with, and contribute to, small-group activities is an indication of a Trainee who has progressed further along the path towards full professional autonomy.

In the Course Organisers' book, outstanding Trainees "contribute to and appreciate the value of group work". They can demonstrate both "leadership" and "the ability to function in teams". They are "supportive to other group members". While they "can use the group to discover their own personal agenda", they "do not exploit the other members of the group to gratify their own emotional needs". Lack of 'group-ability' is indicated by "poor attendance" and "being disruptive in the group". Poorer Trainees "need coercion to participate", are "non-contributory", "cold", "stand-offish" and "isolated". They tend to "use the group to work through their own psychological agenda".

Personal qualities (30%)

Well, we're all only human, aren't we? We like to work with people we like. Amongst the personal characteristics associated with excellence are: "a sense of humour", "affability", "cheerfulness", "conscientiousness", "being good fun", "possessing natural leadership", "enjoying people", "maturity", "willingness to lend a hand", "being tolerant of different attitudes", "serenity", "presence", "fire in the belly" and "a neat dress sense"! "Being isolated and introverted" and "poor personal hygiene" were turn-offs.

Educability (29%)

By what I have termed 'educability' the Course Organisers mean "the ability to grasp and benefit from educational opportunities". The more sophisticated Trainees are "educationally self-directing", liking to "take charge of their own education" and displaying "a continued interest in learning". They are "self-questioning" and "willing to change", "can learn from their mistakes and from traumatic experiences", and "can make use of constructive criticism".

In contrast, the less successful Trainees "have to be spoon-fed". They "lack confidence in their own abilities" and "are undermined by criticism". Their teachers are unable to "instil humility without a loss of confidence".

Considering that Trainers and Course Organisers are paid to promote change in their Trainees, it is perhaps a little surprising to find that the possibility of change ever occurring, especially attitudinal change, is seriously questioned. Yet most of the Course Organisers' gloom about their work reflects ambivalence about whether significant change might not be, at the end of the day, an illusion.

In decreasing order of negativism, here are some of the Course Organisers' more pessimistic views:

"Attitudes are not susceptible to change by education."

"It is impossible to identify or quantify specific areas of teaching that change attitudes."

"My lot never really demonstrated any potential or interest, so there was no question of them fulfilling it!"

"There are real limits to the attainments of an individual which no amount of education will expand; and these limits have to all practical purposes been set before a Trainee embarks on Vocational Training."

"People change their attitudes mainly by cross-fertilization and osmosis, rather than by specific educational efforts."

"Professional growth and attitudinal change only occur as by-products of our teaching of knowledge and skills."

"I try to pull people along, rather than push. You can't instil educational commitment if it's not there. If they refuse to budge, I carry on without them."

"I'm not sure I can do more than sensitize and awaken innate skills."

"I doubt if any course does more than open doors already unlocked."

"By the time I get them, it's too late to change them. Having said that, I think setting an example probably influences them for the better."

One respondent, however, dared to look in the mirror and wrote, "Your study may provide more information about the attitudes of Course Organisers than about Trainees'."

Motivation (28%)

Outstanding Trainees are usually "enthusiastic", "committed" and "eager to learn". The disappointments come from those who are "unmotivated", who "make no effort", and who are "unwilling to involve themselves with their hearts".

It is arguable whether motivation is a separate parameter from, say, response to novelty, educability or mission (see below). Nevertheless, motivation features so prominently in the vocabulary of the Course Organisers that it deserves to be flagged as an issue in its own right.

Balance (20%)

A widely-held belief is that "you can't be a good doctor if you don't achieve a balance between your professional and your private life". Outstanding Trainees seem "personally well-organised" and have "stability in their lives", often in the form of "a supportive spouse". Conversely, some under-achieving Trainees seem to have "poor boundaries", and find that "their energy is sapped by domestic or marital problems". One Course Organiser described how a Trainee had been "too willing to do anything for anyone at any time for his own good".

Industry (19%)

Course Organisers go for Trainees who are "hard-working", ("but uncomplaining"), and who "work hard at whatever job they're in". Such Trainees tend to "do projects and original work". They are "doers, not just full of empty words". Poorer Trainees are described as "work-shy" "clock-watchers", who are "only time-serving".

Communication skills (16%)

Effectiveness at communicating with patients and colleagues is valued, but interestingly was only mentioned by 16% of respondents, who used phrases like "good at interpersonal relationships" or "good communication and consultation skills". "Unwillingness to listen" was criticised, as was the " too laid-back consulting style" of one Trainee, who was "poor at giving structure or confronting when necessary".

Mission (15%)

In the study of successful entrepreneurs by Garfield previously referred to, a sense of 'mission' – a clear and detailed vision of what a person wants out of life – was reckoned to be the source of the peak performance that set priorities, determined behaviour and fuelled motivation. In his view, mission is the cardinal hallmark of excellence. It is also recognised as an important characteristic of excellence in vocational Trainees, though apparently, at only 15%, by a minority of Course Organisers.

Those who acknowledged this quality described it thus:

"Knows where he's going";

"Oriented towards long-term goals";

"Can define personal philosophy, and can apply it simply, objectively, and with determination";

"Has the will to strive towards optimum standards";

"Sustained by personal faith".

Others complained of a "lack of definite aims" or a "laissez-faire attitude to work and life". Some Trainees leave their "good intentions unfulfilled – especially true of men!". One Course Organiser sighed, "Under-achievers seem to me to have lost the ambition to be really good, and are prepared to settle for a comfortable life-style"; and then confessed, "I can't really blame them, either!"

On a positive note, one respondent wrote, "I try to encourage Trainees to 'dream' about the sort of practice they want to work in. I hope this gives them sufficient skills to improve that practice when they get there". Another listed his 'Ideals' – characteristics of an ideal Trainee which included, amongst others:

"Seeks freedom and independence",

"Admires and encourages individual achievement in self and others",

"Orients around an Aristotelian philosophy that holds the individual as the supreme being",

"Orientated towards long-range value-producing goals".

Critical ability (7%)

Under this head are included the abilities to "marshal facts", to "argue a case articulately", and to "establish priorities".

Diversity (7%)

The energy of Trainees regarded as outstanding often spills over into contexts, medical and non-medical, beyond the confines of their current post. They "have experience of a wider world outside medicine"; some have been "committed to working for nuclear disarmament", and others "help famine victims in the third world". They also tend to have "wide-ranging social interests".

THE ICARUS FACTOR

These, then, are the qualities identified by Britain's Course Organisers as the hallmarks of excellence in Vocational Trainees. As descriptions of an ideal, they can probably serve as an educational 'mission statement'. It has become apparent, however, that even as we clarify our vision of the idealised end-result we are faced with a terrible and undermining doubt: can we *teach* these things? We know that some fortunate Trainees at the end of their apprenticeship appear to bear these hallmarks. But are they in fact *teachable*? Two and a half millenia later, we confront the same questions that Meno asked of Socrates: "Is virtue something that can be taught? Or does it come by practice? Or is it neither teaching nor practice that gives it to a man but natural aptitude?"

It is often the case when Trainers and Course Organisers discuss these questions, as they frequently do, that debate degenerates into a 'tis-'tisn't does-doesn't kind of argument, with no satisfactory resolution. Now as a general principle, if the question you are asking produces a silly answer, it's worth asking a different question. So let's try that.

A case can be made for the qualities of excellence to be thought of not as specific educational objectives but as epiphenomena; that is, incidental by-products of an educational environment that has allowed the pupil's natural tendency for self-development to flower unstunted. What we take for excellence is an indication that successful learning is *already* occurring.

The hallmarks of excellence are the vital signs, the temperature, pulse and blood pressure of a living process, a pupil's outward signals that he or she is experiencing an education that is *already* successfully supplying, whether the teacher knows it or not, exactly what is needed. The potential is already there; circumstances can release it. This of course was Socrates' response to Meno, made vivid by the demonstration of the slave's unsuspected intuitive grasp of geometry which could be revealed by skilled questioning. The Trainee is pregnant with pre-resident excellence to which the accomplished teacher can play midwife. A small but extremely significant shift is now implied for the role of teacher. To change the analogy: the difference required of an 'excellence-releasing' teacher is like the difference between driving manual and automatic cars. With a manual car, no forward movement occurs unless the driver exerts pressure on the accelerator; without this, under load the engine stalls. With automatic transmission, the vehicle's impulse is to move inexorably forwards. The driver can regulate this movement with throttle and brake, and even bring it to a temporary halt, but still the vehicle's natural tendency is to be ever moving onwards.

I need a name for this force, this automatic impulse for learners to be ever moving towards their own personal versions of excellence. Because of the obvious associations, let's call it 'the Icarus factor'.

For teachers, trust – trust in the Icarus factor – may prove a greater virtue than control. The teacher's task-defining question has to change. No longer is it a question of "How on earth can I instil excellence?" The teacher needs to ask instead, "How can I create a learning environment where the release of native excellence can take place freely, without distortion or inhibition? Is there anything I might inadvertently be doing which is frustrating my pupil's natural development?" It seems that the pursuit of excellence calls for a clear vision, a clear sense of mission, and a clearing away of obstacles. To teach in these areas means to stimulate, to allow, and then – to get out of the pupil's way.

We can in hindsight spot – and indeed have already discussed – many of the problems which contributed to the sad fate of Icarus as he attempted to soar on his heat-vulnerable wings. But it wasn't the heat that did for Icarus. It wasn't the Icarus factor. It was the shoddy way Daedalus constructed the aerofoils, and the oppressively didactic instructions he gave. What should he have done differently? What difference might have made a difference? Let's see if we can find an answer in teaching terms to the question, "What is the difference that makes the difference?" [4].

Chapter 4

The difference that makes the difference

Not everything that counts can be counted, and not everything that can be counted counts. [1]

FOURTEEN INTO THREE WON'T GO

Vocational Training has thrown a gauntlet at its own feet. The professional excellence we should like our Trainees to aspire to is recognisable, describable, definable in terms of the handful of attributes listed in the previous chapter. I've also suggested (on admittedly only anecdotal evidence so far) that there is an 'Icarus factor' – an intrinsic drive people have, circumstances being propitious, to make the most of themselves and let their natural excellence shine through. Some fortunate individuals make notable progress towards this ideal in the course of their professional apprenticeships, whereas others seem more erratic and in need of guidance. Very well. The task should be easy. We have, in the Educational Paradigm (see Figure 1.1, page 20), a rigorous method for converting general goals into measurably improved performance. Furthermore, it has been found helpful to subdivide the great array of competences needed in general practice into the familiar trinity of Knowledge, Skills and Attitudes. Indeed, so universally and unquestioningly is 'KnowledgeSkillsandAttitudes' held in veneration that, in the reflex facility with which the phrase falls from their tongues, medical teachers today sound like a congregation in more spiritual times professing faith in that other Trinity – Father, Son and Holy Ghost.

So let's see whether the orthodox educational paradigm can accommodate our 14 hallmarks of excellence. Let's first see under which of the three heads of the trinity each of the 14 is best assigned. What will come under '*Knowledge*'? Quite a lot of what makes up 'clinical competence', certainly, and some 'communication skills' of the more mechanical kind;

but not a lot else. How about '*Skills*'? Here we can include the remainder of 'clinical competence', some further 'communication skills', and perhaps 'critical ability', insofar as that consists of the intellectual skills of logical appraisal and evaluation. So the rest ought to count as '*Attitudes*'. Let's see: 'Industry'? Yes; being willing to make an effort, that's probably an attitude. 'Caritas'? Yes. 'Balance' between professional and private life? Yes. 'Motivation' (whatever that means)? Yes. 'Response to novelty'? Not so sure. To be interested in new ideas, and more importantly to follow them up and internalise them, is rather more than an attitude. I'd say the same about 'Self-awareness' too. Recognition of the worth of self-awareness I'd call an attitude, but undertaking systematic cultivation of self-awareness, following it through, and resolving the consequent issues and dilemmas is again something more deep-going than what we normally think of as an attitude.

What's left? A significant residuum of desirable attributes – 'Group-ability', 'Mission', 'Diversity', 'Educability', and a whole range of 'Personal qualities' including curiosity, leadership, kindness, enthusiasm – will simply not fit neatly and comfortably into the bran-tub labelled 'Attitudes'. And even if they did, and we were to try teaching them using the orthodox cycle of Objectives / Teaching strategies / Assessment? What should we be letting ourselves in for? Objectives: "The Trainee shall describe five cases in which patient care was compromised by his or her own psychological hang-ups." Strategies: "Today's tutorial is intended to help you contribute to group work. If you'd just put on these cricket flannels . . ." Or Assessment: "I want to see whether you are undermined by criticism. So switch on the video camera and I'll start to insult you."

Hmmmm! It's not working. There is a problem, and it's caused by trying to coerce excellence into an educational paradigm manifestly too small to accommodate it. If the hallmarks of excellence are treated as educational objectives in the traditional sense, we are immediately condemned to the absurd and ultimately frustrating task of devising assessment tools for highly sensitive and precious human qualities, and making them one by one the targets of a series of artificial teaching strategies. For this reason we have never felt happy about the teaching of attitudes. Attitudes have a 'keep off the grass', 'out of bounds and out of reach' feel to them. We recognise their importance, know them when we see them, and frequently discuss them behind our Trainees' backs (but only in moments of rare bravery to their faces). But we shrink from trying to change them, knowing that the attempt would probably be embarrassing and the results unreliable. So we concentrate on teaching knowledge and skills, which are safer, and just hope for the best as far as the higher-order goals are concerned. Paradoxically – clinical knowledge and skills apart, and I know that's a big exception – it seems that we teach least effectively what most needs learning, and value most highly qualities that are hardest to change.

The most useful lessons our Trainees could possibly learn are the ones we don't know how to teach; yet we're paid instructors! Small wonder the Course Organisers who replied to my questionnaire were prey to doubts about the worth of their role. Time and again the ambivalent message came – measuring and modifying attitudes is (a) hard work, (b) probably impossible, and (c) something they would like to be better at. And although they knew that excellence beckoned like a high and sunlit canopy of great trees, they felt that reality consisted all too often of hacking away in gloomy thickets at ground level.

We have reached *aporia* – that helplessness, confusion and disillusion familiar to the interlocutors of Socrates when the foundations of their apparent wisdom subsided beneath their feet. We have been touched by the sting-ray. And I say, "Good!" Disenchantment with rigid educational method is the appropriate and necessary response. Let's now find a way forward. What would Socrates do? He would ask an awareness-raising question. So let's ask ourselves, "What is our attitude to attitudes?" We have attitudes about the word 'attitude', and about the concept of an attitude, and they're not very helpful. So I suggest we dispense with them.

"ATTITUDES SHOULD BE ABOLISHED"

The word 'attitude' has become, because of its negative associations, the Vocational Training equivalent of the demoralising 'fat folder' patient in general practice, in prospect whereof the heart sinks. Talk of 'attitudes' intimidates us, paralyses thought, and legitimises feelings of impotence. When the word is mentioned at all it's usually in the context of an 'attitude problem':

– "I don't like your attitude";
– "You're going to have to change your attitude";
– "That's the wrong attitude";
– "What kind of attitude's that?";
– "Don't take that attitude!"

We shouldn't underestimate the power of word association. 'Knowledge' and 'skill' sound like desirable commodities, things it would be nice to have in abundance, positive and legitimate training goals. But who the hell wants 'attitudes'?

So let's stop talking in terms of 'attitudes'. Let's instead use the words 'values' and 'beliefs'.

This substitution is more than a mere semantic nicety. 'Values' and 'beliefs' have much more positive associations. They sound precious and interesting. We can discuss values and beliefs with greater optimism, and without feeling the same helplessness or discouragement that talk of attitudes reflexly induces. Thinking not of people's attitudes but of their values and beliefs will free us from some limiting reactions, and will open up some difficult territory to understanding and intervention.

What's the difference? Essentially it's a question of ownership. 'Values' and 'beliefs' are parts of your mental furniture that *you know you have*. Your personal history, your background and upbringing have created for you belief-systems and value-systems with which you feel a strong sense of identification. They make perfect sense *for* you and *of* you. 'Attitudes' on the other hand are inferences drawn by someone else. Attitudes are what *I think you have*. I see the things you do and hear the things you say, and infer from them that you have a particular attitude. But because it is I who have drawn the inference, the attributes I ascribe to you are contaminated by my own perceptual mechanisms. I may well have misperceived you; and because I only know a fraction of your true depth and complexity, I probably misunderstand you. From a subjective point of view, I know I have certain beliefs and values – they're mine. But I don't feel as if I have attitudes. I don't *own* them.

There are some immediate educational advantages to be gained from talking of values and beliefs rather than of attitudes. Firstly, values and beliefs can be identified with potentially much greater accuracy, being free of observer bias. Secondly, because they arise from personal experience, beliefs and values can be expanded or modified by fresh experience. Since value systems make perfect sense to the owner, then provided the sense of ownership is maintained, any development of them also makes perfect sense and is therefore imbued with commitment and motivational energy.

It's going to be my contention that non-judgemental awareness of as many as possible of both Trainee's and Trainer's beliefs and values is an effective catalyst for constructive change within their relationship. Techniques for increasing non-judgemental awareness of values will prove effective teaching tools. When an individual's beliefs and values are aligned with opportunities in the educational environment, the results are growth, development and motivation. If on the other hand circumstance or experience are, without being recognised, at odds with currently held values, the resultant misalignment produces tension and under-achievement.

THE PSYCHOBIOLOGY OF BELIEFS, VALUES AND MISSION

Like all components of systems which are organically or psychologically alive, beliefs and values have their place in the overall functioning. It will help us now to develop a sense of the roles played by beliefs and values in maintaining mental homeostasis and in stimulating the flow of motivational energy.

Life, both physical and mental, is the temporary advantage of stability over entropy, of adaptation over disintegration. Things are forever happening which, did we not learn to do something about them, would get the better of us. Beliefs and values are to mental life what anatomy and physiology are to that of the body – semi-permanent links, formed by processes of natural selection, between the evolutionary legacy of the distant past and the repertoire of responses needed to survive the future. Within the life-span of an individual mind, beliefs and value-systems form a cognitive bridge between a person's past – his or her cultural background and life events – and the future he or she endeavours through education and determination to create.

Beliefs

Remember how in the first chapter of this book we distinguished between the deep structure of our total experience and the simplified surface structures in which we encode sufficient of its detail to get by on a day-to-day basis? Beliefs are surface structures – 'good enough to get by with' working summaries of everything we learned during our formative years. Beliefs are what we are left with when we combine the infinities of our personal life-stories with our nervous system's tendency to reduce the world's complexity down to manageable over-simplifications. They are the bets we make with ourselves that, "in our experience", particular types of things will turn out to have particular properties or behave in particular ways. Beliefs are probability statements crediting an object or event with particular enduring attributes, so that the next time we meet it we don't have to stop to reassess, but can get straight on with responding. Reaction time is thereby saved, and as long as no contrary evidence is encountered, the belief is reinforced. An example or two will make this clearer.

I'm an only child, and, as luck would have it, I've never yet knowingly been in circumstances where having a sibling would have been invaluable. I'm also single. I condense these accidents of history down into a belief that I'm self-reliant: that is, at the moment I believe, with a *probability* of about 90%, that I (the *object*) have the *attribute* of self-reliance. Events could occur such as the loss of family or friends or falling unexpectedly in love, that would reduce that probability, even below 50% where the opposite belief, that I'm not self-reliant after all, may come to predominate. But for the time being, till fresh evidence shows up, I'll keep believing.

Because our beliefs are in such constant daily rehearsal it seldom occurs to us to re-examine their source in past experiences, which although formative may have been arbitrary or misleading. The aging memories of once-crucial events lie undisturbed like furniture in a locked room in a seldom-visited wing of mind's mansion, shadowed by the drawn curtains of a defensive forgetfulness and covered over by the dust-sheets of passing time. In this musty gloom it takes either the very determined or the very unexpected to let in the light and prompt a bout of spring-cleaning. Here's a true story.

Over twenty years ago a young man called, let's say, Lance, lived through a soap opera of painful family circumstances. As a result Lance developed a constellation of beliefs about himself and his destiny, all of them self-deprecating. He believed that he had been irretrievably damaged; that he was alone and unsupported; that he had to struggle to achieve any sort of recognition, and that no matter what he achieved it wouldn't be enough to win him lasting approval or affection. Over the intervening years Lance has nonetheless achieved a significant measure of academic and creative success, which has to some degree challenged and recast what he believes about himself. And yet, and yet . . . He told me recently how he had been to see the film *Music Box*. In the film an aging and likeable Hungarian immigrant to the USA is unexpectedly, forty years on, accused of war crimes against the Jews in Budapest. His adoring lawyer daughter successfully defends him on grounds of mistaken identity. But just as his innocence is proclaimed she finds incontrovertible evidence of his guilt. The father she believed a paragon turns out to be a beast, and because she also believes in justice she denounces him. Lance was profoundly unsettled by this story. He identified with – no, recognised; no, remembered – the sense of betrayal and abandonment in the film's closing sequences. It restimulated his own desolation when as a teenager he had discovered his own father – the one parent who had shown him some affection – in an act of incest, and had reluctantly denounced him. Lance had been both betrayer and betrayed; the family had closed ranks around the father, leaving Lance feeling isolated, alienated and orphaned. Then, twenty years on, a vivid story on a screen sneaks past his carefully constructed defences, which is the point of stories, and reminds him unexpectedly of events that, far from being psychologically dead, are in fact alive in his everyday thoughts, feelings and beliefs. This insight offers another chance to rid his injurious belief-system of its illusory truth and permanence. He has the freedom now to accept the validity of the more self-enhancing events of his later life. In other words, he has been rendered free to learn. Again that echoing line of Bachelard:

But the image has touched the depths before it stirs the surface.

Values

Beliefs are massive but also shy creatures, like whales, and Bachelard's 'depths' are their natural habitat in the ocean of the psyche. That ocean can only sustain a smallish population of serious beliefs; on the surface, where most of life is lived, we prefer to view beliefs from a distance, finding them a little too overpowering close up. In everyday transactions, 'values' are more in evidence than beliefs. Values are more like dolphins than whales. More plentiful and less ponderous than beliefs, values inhabit the surface waters of mental life, leaping every now and then into full conscious awareness before falling back into the warm waters of the only-just-subconscious.

It will do no harm to spend a moment anticipating where this talk of values will lead us. It became clear to me from studying the replies of the Course Organisers to my survey that a Traineeship's educational destiny – the extent to which the accomplishments of its autumnal phase exceeded, matched up to or fell short of the promise of its spring – depended less on the minutiae of knowledge and skills acquired along the way and more on the degree to which Trainer and Trainee came to develop mutual regard for each other's personal and professional values. While the claim, "Get the values right and the education will look after itself" is certainly an over-simplification, I would submit that a Traineeship where the value-systems of the participants are mutually appreciated and substantially in alignment is a more fulfilling and altogether more responsive Traineeship. Value-congruence in a Traineeship is like power-assisted steering in a car – it only needs fingertip pressure on the steering wheel, and manoeuvring in tight spaces is much easier.

It began to look as if 'the difference that makes the difference' might lie in our ability as teachers so to structure our Trainees' educational environment that the maturing of their value systems is enhanced with as much reliability as the acquisition of specific knowledge and skills. So I found myself wondering how people come by the sorts of values which sometimes prove conflictual in Traineeships; what function values serve in conditioning people's responses to the multiplicity of educational opportunities that come their way; and whether it is possible to establish points of potential leverage upon the relevant value systems, so that change can be brought about in an ethical and effective way.

I've already quoted the Zen saying that goes, "When the pupil is ready, the master appears". Waking earlier than usual one Sunday I turned on the bedside radio and caught a repeat of an Open University broadcast on 'Living with Technology'. Stephen Cotgrove, Professor of Sociology at the University of Bath, was explaining how the controversy surrounding issues such as nuclear power or environmentalism indicated a conflict not of information but of the values held by opposing groups. Although opponents belaboured each other with what each claimed were 'facts', they were in truth brandishing their own cultural values in a kind of tribal loyalty from which argument would not and could not dissuade them. I jotted down what I took to be the talk's conclusion: 'It's circumstances, not arguments, that change values'.

I corresponded with Professor Cotgrove who, although by then retired, invited me to meet him. Our discussion confirmed for me the importance of searching beneath surface issues for the core values and beliefs that are at stake when people of apparently equal sincerity find themselves in passionate disagreement. (Wouldn't it be a relief if this principle were better appreciated by the politicians who forever bad-mouth each other, and by those who interview them for the media?) In the Preface to one of his books, Cotgrove writes, ' . . . central to any understanding of change (are) the values and goals to which groups in society attach importance and which they come to define as a basis for legitimate . . . demands' [2]. Cotgrove's work also showed how, for all their highly personal and sensitive nature, values can be identified and quantified for research purposes by the careful construction of rating scales using value-free language and factor analysis.

Sociologists tell us that values are 'bipolar judgements': that is, we either like or dislike something; we rate it either good or bad; we are for it or against it. Value judgements can be attached to objects, or concepts, or people, or events, or behaviours or thoughts – and the effect of making a value judgement about something is that we are subsequently predisposed to behave *consistently* towards it. The strength and persistence of that predisposition are measures of the intensity of the value judgement in question. The consistent nature of value-driven behaviour provides some stability and predictability in our responses to a turbulent and often dangerous world. Values are therefore part of a behavioural auto-pilot, with a Darwinian pay-off in terms of social survival.

All this boils down to is that, because of our past experience and the beliefs we have extracted from it, we value certain attributes in preference to others; this saves us having to think too much about every least little dilemma. The importance of this piece of common sense lies in its potential to bring within educational reach those occasions when the entrenched nature of certain values becomes a liability rather than an asset.

We quite like to camouflage our values. But they give themselves away. Values lie hidden in a thousand judgement-inflected nuances of everyday speech. Values are to be found in our "obviously"s and "of course"s, our "never"s and our "always"; in our assumings and presumings and supposings; in our starting positions and basic principles; in my "insight", your "guess" and his "sheer fluke"; in all the things we take for granted, and the things we take pride in, and the things we take umbrage at; in the things we've always dreamed of and the things we'd never have dreamed; in the foibles of our friends and the follies of our foes. But perhaps most importantly, our values can be flushed from cover whenever we have to make choices.

Another unexpected master appeared – this time Robert McKee, a Hollywood teacher of screen-writing who presents a fascinating three-day workshop on story structure. What (McKee asked rhetorically) does a film audience want? They want to discover something important about themselves, and to discover it in ways that surprise and move them. How are they to do this? By identifying with a character they care about. How do they identify with a character? By seeing a hero or heroine, with needs and frailties such as we all have, pursuing, through a series of reversals, some goal that matters. How do they get to care about what happens to the protagonist? By discovering more and more depth to the character as the story unfolds. What's depth in a character? The gradual revelation of the real values his or her life is lived by. And how do you tell the real values people live their lives by? By the choices they make under pressure.

Our values are revealed by the choices we make under pressure. In effect, values *are* the choices people make under pressure. There are of course degrees of pressure, but the mildest and the weightiest alike provoke value-imbued choices. Two housewives want to make ice-cubes in the freezer. One uses disposable polythene former-bags, because she values her own convenience; the other uses a conventional ice-tray, because she values environment-friendliness more. Two old men within days of death from stomach cancer are being nursed by their wives. One wife, who has always valued their open and honest relationship, talks freely with her husband about his approaching death and her own widowhood. The other, who knows how a show of emotion has always embarrassed her husband, so values his right to die in his own way that she talks through pretended smiles of a recovery neither believes in. Same situations, different values, different choices under pressure, explicable not in terms of right or wrong but by reference to the antecedent life events and the beliefs distilled from them.

In the film *The Karate Kid* which I've already referred to, young Danny spots and fancies Ali. She is teased by the Cobra gang; Danny has to choose whether or not to intervene on her behalf. He intervenes, and we thereby learn that he values loyalty (or maybe sex) more than his own personal safety. The Cobras beat him up; what is he to do about it? Danny must now choose between the rival values of pacifism and the use of force. He chooses force, specifically karate, showing us that he values self-discipline as well. Later, when Mr Miyagi the karate master agrees to teach him, one particular sequence of scenes graphically reveals some of the values underlying the relationship of tutelage. Danny's first lessons consist of cleaning endless cars and polishing vast areas of wooden flooring. Danny, who thinks he's being exploited, has to choose whether or not to come back for further 'lessons'. Back he comes, and so we learn that he puts more value on trust and friendship and the chance to learn than on personal convenience. Next Miyagi tells the increasingly reluctant Danny to paint the fence, and now Miyagi's own values are on the line. He has to choose between increasing the pressure on Danny (and risking losing his pupil), and relaxing the pressure and losing the chance of maximal teaching impact. Miyagi values the 'teacher' role more than the 'nice guy' role – Danny must next paint the house. Danny, who by now has committed himself to obedience, is at the point of Socratic aporia where things no longer make any sense. "I don't believe this", he cries. "I'm going home!" Miyagi, a true disciple of Socrates, values insight above instruction. He shows Danny how the circular arm movements he has practised in the cleaning and polishing, and the up-and-down and side-to-side wrist movements of the painting, and which are now thoroughly ingrained, are in fact the essential reflexes of karate. Danny has been well taught, better taught than he or we realised at the time. Appreciation of the lesson is all the greater for its having been delayed and disguised. We the audience have discovered something important about learning, and have discovered it in ways that surprise and move us.

So – values are a feature of mental architecture whose purpose is to inform our decision-making so that it accords with what we believe, and to provide a sense of consistency and purpose when we consider our options. Our values are found in the honest answers we might give if the little voice of consciousness inside our heads kept asking, "Why am I doing this?"

Where do we get our values from? Values, as we have seen, are beliefs chunked down for application at a single decision-point, and beliefs are the condensations of what events have so far taught us. So, just as we have intentional control over some but not all of the things that happen to us, we can intentionally control some but not all of our values. Many values are directly handed down to us from the significant adults in our formative years, (or 'parents' as they used to be called). Barring major trauma, most of us believe that the values of the environment that nurtured us – people, culture, events – are, since we have come through so far relatively unscathed, the 'right' ones. It may be our good fortune so far not to have met circumstances that significantly challenge them. If, however, we should find ourselves in situations with which our existing values are incompatible, change of some kind is inevitable. We may by an act of conscious choice change our values, as when for instance the child of an alcoholic decides on life-long abstemiousness. Or we may compromise, as a parent badly beaten in childhood compromises when he "never takes a belt" to his own children, "just the flat of my hand". Another thing we often do with incompatible values is just tolerate the incompatibility: we seem able quite happily to compartmentalise this aspect of our personalities, behaving true to one professed value on one occasion and to another, quite contradictory, at another. The world may call this inconsistency or hypocrisy; we prefer to think of ourselves as "complex characters" who are "only human, after all". But value-conflicts should perhaps ideally be resolved by learning – taking the risk of making a different choice under pressure, seeing whether in fact it might not turn out to be a better one, and allowing a shift in values that increases our behavioural options in future.

We have seen how, confronted with a choice, we invoke a value. Of great educational significance, however, is the corollary: *if you want to identify a value, present a choice*. The tactical importance of this will become clearer when in Chapter 9 we look at techniques for identifying and resolving value-conflicts.

Most of what has so far been said about the psychobiological function of values has emphasised their role in stabilising our sense of personal identity through life's vicissitudes. Values have a second role, also potentially of great educational power: they make it possible to set *goals* for ourselves. As well as being reactive, values also become *proactive*. If we value certain things highly enough we don't wait around until they happen to turn up; we proactively seek them out. The really important and powerful values don't merely select options – they go out and grab them. Opportunities aren't just seized – they're created. When values acquire the motivational energy to make things happen, and carve out a path towards our personal goals in a sustained and coordinated way, they take on a role best conveyed by the term *'mission'*.

Mission

A sense of 'mission', although it featured as one of our 14 hallmarks of excellence, isn't something we like to dwell on in British professional training. It sounds either too evangelical or too transatlantic. But all mission means in this context is having a clear and abiding idea of the kind of doctor we might be, and the types of things we might do, that would most completely honour the values we most dearly cherish. Mission is values which have become articulated and focussed – a detailed blueprint of an idealised future self, a plan for achieving congruence between the aspirations of the life within and the realities of the life external. Mission serves as a motivational power-house for selecting, creating and implementing educational opportunities which contribute to the mission. The importance of mission, as we shall see, is clearly acknowledged in sporting and commercial worlds. The more clearly an end-point can be visualised, the more likely it is to be achieved. 'Target' and 'ambition' need not be dirty words: creating the mental possibility of fulfilment is halfway to creating the reality. The imagining renders more likely the coming-to-pass.

There's an excellent little cameo study of mission in – you guessed it – *The Karate Kid*. (You'll really *have* to get this film, a fine allegory about apprenticeship, out of the video library!)

Mr Miyagi, the handyman who happens to be a karate master, has mended Danny's bike. Danny calls round to thank him and finds Miyagi trimming and shaping his miniature *bonsai* trees with evident skill. Danny becomes curious and asks, "Are those real trees?"

Miyagi:	You like see? Come inside.
Danny:	How'd they get so small?
Miyagi:	I train. Clip here, tie there.
Danny:	Did you go to school for this?

Miyagi: No. Father teach.

Danny: He a gardener?

Miyagi: No, fisherman.

Danny: These are really beautiful.

Miyagi: Come. You try.

Danny: No no, I don't know how to do this stuff. I don't want to
              mess it up.

Miyagi: Sit down.
              (Danny settles himself before an untrimmed pine specimen.)
              Close eye. Trust.
              Concentrate. Think only – *tree*.
              Think of perfect picture, down to last pine-needle. Wipe
              mind clean of everything but – *tree*. Nothing exist whole
              world, only – *tree*.
              You got it?
              (Danny nods.)
              Open eye. Remember picture?
              (Danny nods again. Miyagi hands him the hasami, *the bonsai-
              pruning secateurs.)*
              Make like picture.
              Just trust picture.

Danny: How do I know if my picture's the right one?

Miyagi: If come from inside you – *always* right one.

A clear sense of professional mission has a number of desirable spin-offs for
the educational process. Perhaps the most important is that mission can
motivate. The Trainee whose chosen professional role allows the expression of important beliefs and values, and who finds these broadly in
alignment with the beliefs and values pervading the educational environment, is a motivated Trainee. Furthermore, mission is the strategic force
giving overall direction and purpose to the long-term trajectory of a
Traineeship. Mission provides the point; it answers the questions,
"What's my aim in doing this? Is it what I want? How does this fit in?
Where's it leading? What do I need to do next?" Mission, in George
Bernard Shaw's phrase, is 'a purpose recognised by yourself as a mighty
one.'

Values create mission, and mission shapes trajectory. Within the trajectory of a Traineeship a long succession of learning opportunities will
present themselves: awareness of a Trainee's personal mission allows

teacher and pupil to assign priorities and make choices. Learning that respects the pupil's current values and sense of mission produces the longest-lasting and most appreciated changes in behaviour. As Figure 4.1 indicates, new knowledge and behaviour in their turn become part of the ever-increasing accumulation of experience. This in due course produces new generations of upgraded beliefs and values and continuing refinements of mission.

In this sense, value-congruent learning is a psychobiological process. Cognitive growth and personality development are the results of interaction between slowly-evolving internal variables – beliefs, values and mission – and the learning opportunities encountered in the educational environment. A process akin to natural selection operates. By and large, those learning outcomes which increase the adaptive usefulness of the learner's belief- and value-systems in the real world are the ones that survive. What we call 'motivation' and 'excellence' are physical signs that this homeostatic learning process is at work, just as a stable blood pressure indicates functional integrity of the circulatory system.

Later chapters of this book will address more rigorously the principles and practice of intervening educationally so as to maximise learning efficiency. My main purpose in this chapter has been to establish that motivation and excellence are not optional afterthoughts or mysterious 'gifts from the gods', but are the inevitable outcomes of an educational experience that understands the central role of values in determining what and how an individual learns.

THE E-ZONE

We are now in a position to suggest wherein lies the educational 'difference that makes the difference'.

In postgraduate professional education, three balls – three independent variables – are to be juggled. They are, not necessarily in order of importance:

– Curriculum,
– Mission, and
– Educational opportunities.

Firstly, the discipline imposes its own curricular requirements. In General Practice these are well documented and have been referred to already. An education that neglects the core of appropriate knowledge and skills sells short all concerned. There is a certain corpus of expertise that is required of a independent practitioner, regardless of how it is acquired and

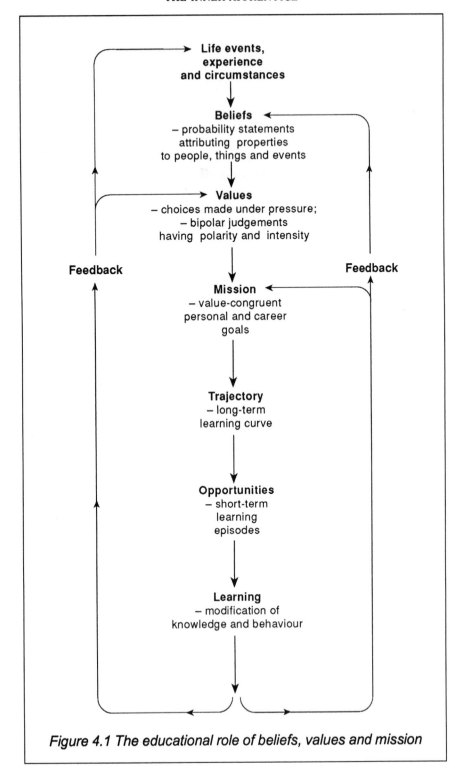

Figure 4.1 The educational role of beliefs, values and mission

whether the Trainee enjoys it or not. Secondly, each individual Trainee brings to the Traineeship his or her own personal learning agenda – a pre-existing set of beliefs and values derived from past experience, and a mission (explicit or latent) which will consolidate and develop them. The Trainee's learning goals may or may not coincide with the requirements of curriculum, but, as we have seen, it is mission rather than curriculum that motivates change. Finally, Traineeships differ in the degree to which they supply the opportunities required either by curriculum or by mission. There may be a superfluity or a dearth of appropriate tuition; there may be blind spots or hobby-horses; or there may be no shortage of good intention but rather a lack of relevant teaching skills, so that needs are not matched by corresponding resources.

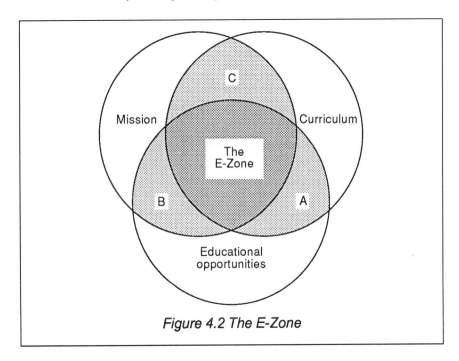

Figure 4.2 The E-Zone

Figure 4.2 shows graphically, in a Venn diagram, how these three variables interact with each other. There are areas where there may be *no* overlap to speak of. The curriculum may contain topics that are neither taught nor cared about. The educational environment may afford opportunities that contribute nothing to the requirements of curriculum or to the personal aspirations of the Trainee. And some of the Trainee's mission goals may have no place in the curriculum, and no need of education to satisfy them.

Of more interest are the areas marked A, B and C in the diagram. Area A, where curriculum overlaps with the educational environment, is the domain of the 'paradigm slaves'. Here all educational effort is directed towards the demands of curriculum, whose requirements are to be met without question or compromise. Because mission is excluded, a Trainee-ship conducted in area A is one that 'goes through the motions'; no-one can say the ground was not covered, but oh! how mechanically and oh! with how little enthusiasm.

Area B, where mission flourishes and opportunities abound but curriculum is neglected, is a potential fool's paradise of collusiveness. If a Trainee whose mission is to be the best golf-playing rheumatologist who never passed a speculum happens to work with a Trainer who loves rheumatology as much as he loves golf and hates gynaecology, the predictable outcome may be fun and may be fulfilling, but will be far from comprehensive. If Area A was the area of paradigm slavery, B is the area of phoney liberation, where rigour, in the name of Trainee-centred learning, is sacrificed to sloth or to a slogan.

Area C depicts the state to which a motivated and discerning Trainee will retreat in the absence of skilled and sensitive teaching. Untutored, mission and curriculum will achieve a measure of reciprocal satisfaction; learning may wither yet not quite die under conditions of educational drought. In the absence of direction, learning is of necessity self-directed. But it's a fine line that divides 'self-directed learning' from unstructured apathy. How much greater could have been the achievement had inclination and requirement been matched by opportunity.

Imagine now a happy state where teaching skills are able to coax into alignment a Trainee's personal aspirations on one hand and the hall-marks of the craft consummately performed on the other. This is the educational Shangri-la where Excellence Emerges – the 'E-Zone'. In the E-Zone the subjective desires of mission and the objective requirements of curriculum coincide, and the means of attaining both are freely available. Motivation is at its most resolute and the drive towards self-fulfilment – the Icarus factor – is most in evidence.

My thesis is this: a teacher who can offer as much constructive intervention in a Trainee's beliefs, values and mission goals as he can in the more familiar demands of curriculum, i.e. who is at home in the E-Zone, is a teacher who can make 'the difference that makes the difference'.

THE DIFFERENCE THAT MAKES THE DIFFERENCE

Excellence can be thought of in terms of the array of values it encapsulates. Glance back for a moment at Figure 3.1 (page 56): the 14 so-called hallmarks of excellence are in fact statements about the set of values a Trainer would like to see installed in his Trainee. A Trainer seeking excellence for his Trainee is in fact establishing a 'curriculum of specific values' in the same way that the conventional educational paradigm sets curricular objectives in the areas of knowledge and skills. Values being the choices made under pressure, the Trainer hopes that the pressure of day-to-day work and learning will lead to a Trainee choosing, for example, curiosity rather than indifference in the face of novel ideas; compassion rather than aloofness in the face of human distress; self-knowledge rather than self-deception; a sense of purpose rather than aimlessness – and so on down the list.

Now that we have seen how beliefs, values and mission have their place in individual psychobiology, contributing to social survival just as organ systems do to physical survival, we can begin to discern where and how a skilled teacher might be able to assist in the maturation of a Trainee's value systems and motivation. Let's recap.

The educational 'difference that makes the difference' is the teacher's ability to supply a learning environment that can set and meet 'value' objectives with as much skill and reliability as 'knowledge and skill' ones. This calls for a number of teaching skills and techniques over and above those usually recognised.

Trust

Teaching in the E-Zone demands several varieties of trust. The teacher needs to trust that we all – teachers and pupils – have greater resources within us than we usually take for granted. The relationship of tutelage is founded on trust – trust that each party will respect both the strengths and insecurities of the other. The best guarantee of this is perhaps to ensure that the traffic in vulnerability is not one-way. Disclosing beliefs and values exposes potential areas of defencelessness, and for a Trainer to demonstrate openness of the "I'll tell you mine if you'll tell me yours" kind is an effective builder of trust.

Identifying beliefs and values

Our belief systems, as we have seen, are the mental legacies of our own personal life stories, interpreted in such a way that the person we find events have made of us can be reassuringly perceived as acceptable, consistent and understandable. In a sense, we *are* our core beliefs: once they are revealed there is no further hiding place to which we can retreat without fundamentally changing our sense of who we are and what we stand for. To expose one's beliefs with complete honesty is to be in a state of psychological undress, which is a lot to ask of anyone, teacher or pupil. This is the terrible challenge confronting the teacher. Modification of a pupil's job-related belief systems is potentially the most precious form of professional education; yet in attempting it the most exquisitely sensitive areas of individuality are apparently threatened.

But just as most people would now acknowledge that modern life is the freer for having shaken off Victorian prudery about sex, death and other no-go areas, we should risk not allowing beliefs and values to remain taboo topics in education. In our roles as doctors we are used to dealing sensitively with tender flesh and fragile psyches. We owe it to our pupils to prove equally skilful physicians to any of their beliefs and values which might stand in the way of their professional well-being. Shirking this admittedly difficult task is a form of unkindness: education towards excellence involves liberation from outmoded and incongruent values at least as much as the inculcation of relevant knowledge and skills.

In accomplishing this, it will be helpful to remember how beliefs and values are components in a psychobiological process analogous to the physiological processes in which our medical training has equipped us to intervene. In principle, beliefs and values are accessible to the familiar and traditional diagnostic approach of taking a full history, carrying out a systematic examination (both general and symptom-specific), and if necessary undertaking special tests. In later sections of this book I'll attempt to translate this generality into practical techniques.

Harnessing values to mission and trajectory

Merely clarifying a Trainee's beliefs and values, and even honing them to (dreadful phrase!) maximum appropriateness is not enough. The loftiest of ideals, if unexpressed in action, result in only 'armchair excellence'. Indeed, the loftier the ideal the greater the risk of dissociation from real life. The teacher who wants to work in the E-Zone is a 'midwife to mission', who can help a pupil bridge a potential inertia gap between aspiration and achievement. Mission is the half-way stage between the two – a clear and motivating vision of a future course of action whereby the strongest beliefs and the most important values are fully expressed. Teaching that can take good intentions and convert them into a well-timed, well-paced and coherent learning trajectory is teaching that helps make the difference. A good teacher can catch a dream and give it a deadline.

Garfield [3] observes how, every day, 'people with no particularly deep purpose achieve a lot of goals. They complete reports; make sales; ship orders; check off everything on their to-do lists. In the short run, those completions feel good. And they gradually fit together to make a trap. If, over time, the people checking off one goal after another do not see their work contributing to a larger pattern and an overall objective, they can develop the treadmill blues. Work begins to feel endlessly repetitive. . . Satisfaction and desire decline. Performance deteriorates.'

These are the 'paradigm slaves'. In the traditional educational paradigm it is the job description and the curriculum it spawns that generate the nitty-gritty of teaching agenda. I challenge this. A job description and its derived goals and objectives can't be relied on to produce sufficient motivating force to keep learning on track and fired up. My contention will be that *mission* should shape a learning trajectory, not curriculum. Mission, in a global sense, provides energy and commitment to the overall trajectory of a Traineeship, and it also sparks off a series of 'sub-missions' which endow successive days, weeks and months with purpose and enthusiasm. Such is the internal wisdom of the Trainee's unconscious learning mechanisms that in hindsight the important parts of the curriculum will be found to have been taken in along the way. Mission really can be entrusted with responsibility for shaping the day-to-day trajectory of learning. This may come as a dangerous renunciation of all the educational theory we have been taught, but it would have been understood and accepted without question by the medieval apprentice-masters. They still have much to teach us.

Effective micro-teaching

Socrates has shown us what many of today's educationists still regard as the epitome of effective teaching on a moment-by-moment timescale. In this book's first chapter, 'On Apprenticeship', we saw how Socrates' skill lay in his mastery of the awareness-raising question, combined with a keen sense of how a pupil's inappropriate beliefs could be rendered wobbly enough to be changeable. These are enviable skills, and, as I hope to show, trainable ones.

Feedback

All learning depends on feedback – the outcome of newly-learned behaviour being afforded the chance to modify subsequent rehearsals of it before it becomes set. Learning to ride a bicycle is a good example of this process operating at a proprioceptive level and on a virtually instantaneous timescale. In another setting and on a slower timescale, everyday clinical practice, feedback is again central to improvement. If my diagnosis or therapeutics is inappropriate, I soon find out – the patient (or the partner next consulted!) will soon tell me. In Vocational Training, the widespread use of formative assessment is another acknowledgement of the pivotal role of feedback in establishing and maintaining useful change, even if its implementation sometimes seems to lack finesse.

However, feedback in the domains of beliefs and values is an altogether more haphazard affair. David Bohm is a quantum physicist of world renown whose originality of thought has enabled him to cross interdisciplinary boundaries with aplomb. In an interview with Ernest Rossi, Bohm makes the point that the human brain is imperfectly equipped to generate and use feedback in the realm of thoughts and ideas [4]. Neural feedback mechanisms are most securely established in the lower-level systems of brain stem, cerebellum and paleo-cortex. But at the higher levels of neo-cortical functioning, our brains seem to generate new behavioural options more quickly than feedback can modify them. We think faster than we can learn. Bohm says:

> The body is set up to know that it has produced a movement via the proprioceptive cues it receives as feedback. However, we cannot distinguish between our self-world-image and some independent reality, especially when our self-world-image is powerful. The older structure of the brain had no reason for distinguishing images from reality. An experience of an image could be taken for an experience of the outer object. This is acceptable for the animal, and perhaps for Stone-Age humans. But it is not acceptable for us now, since our neo-cortex has become involved in such powerful activities.
>
> Consider, for example, the possibilities of nuclear war over subjective conflicts that are mistaken for so-called "objective truth" or "reality". Essentially, the neo-cortex lacks proprioception or appropriate feedback about the relative value of its creations: thoughts, beliefs, images, values, and so forth. If the neo-cortex could perceive the destructive implications of what it was doing, as it does with bodily movement, it would stop immediately.'

Bohm goes on to discuss the strong sense of attachment we feel to our preferred self-image, the result of over-identification with our personal history or cultural background. Accurate self-perception, he says, would require some proper system of feedback to the learning mechanisms of the neo-cortex.

> It is a question of values (he maintains). The word *value* is based on the root word *valor*, meaning strength. Your values give strength to your actions . . . But while the act of valuing is what gives strength, the things that we value may become confused . . . The word *mediocre* has a root meaning "halfway up the mountain". If you are going to climb a high mountain, you have to give it high value. Some people get halfway up and then other values such as comfort and security intervene and stop their progress up the mountain. So they become mediocre. The word *mediocre* unfortunately contains a note of condemnation; it is actually a conflict of values . . . (So if) I've stopped halfway up, I must be giving more value to something else. Then I've got to find what that is, right? The typical things are: "I want to be liked, I want to be comfortable, I want to fit into the consensus." . . . On an unconscious level, we give high value to our old programs.

We are thoroughly familiar with the concept of feedback at biochemical and proprioceptive levels; and we acknowledge the value of formative assessment in providing feedback in the acquisition of knowledge and skills. But in relation to beliefs and values, the bed-rock of professional excellence, educative feedback is often rudimentary. There may be none at all, other than some unprofessional and unhelpful griping about Trainees' shortcomings behind their backs. Or feedback takes an un-constructive and confrontational form, on the lines, "You'll have to buck your ideas up!" Or potentially useful feedback may be so far delayed in time as to lose any relevance. What is needed by the teacher who would be midwife to excellence is a safe and effective way of feeding back to a Trainee the impact of his or her values and beliefs on daily practice in a 'mutative' form – a form that can lead on to intentional change.

THE INNER APPRENTICE

This may sound esoteric, fanciful or altogether too theoretical to be of much use. But it's not. Every teacher has a secret ally, which was planted by nature in the mind of every pupil as spymasters plant 'sleepers' amongst their enemies, waiting patiently and inconspicuously to be called into effective service when the time is right. We all have an 'Inner

Apprentice' – a set of learning mechanisms much more subtle and sophisticated yet at the same time much more familiar than conventional educational theory has acknowledged. The Inner Apprentice learns *everything*, not just facts and skills. The Inner Apprentice is perpetually curious; and to this end it can create and modify beliefs and values, generate motivation, and come up with insights – all in the interest of maintaining our ability to adapt to constant change. In the next chapters, Part III of this book, we shall be getting to know the Inner Apprentice – how and what it learns, and the ways it can communicate with teachers, and they with it. I hope as I develop these ideas that you the reader will often be saying to yourself, "Oh I knew *that!*" Good. There's nothing new or mysterious about the Inner Apprentice. But it would be nice to become better friends with this rather shy creature, and to know how to coax it into better co-operation as we try to provide for our pupils 'the difference that makes the difference'.

Part III
The Inner Apprentice

A patient in psychotherapy told her therapist,

> "You don't begin at the surface – not because you begin at the depth, but because *you* don't begin. You induce beginning in me . . . I know the springboard I need. I know which door I want you to open on my behalf."

(quoted by Cox and Theilgaard in Mutative Metaphors in Psychotherapy)

Chapter 5
The Inner Apprentice

> The Sailor cannot see the North,
> but knows the Needle can.
>
> Emily Dickinson

A paradox lies at the heart of all formal teaching, a paradox which becomes all the more unsettling, for teachers at least, the further we find ourselves along the road from primary and secondary to undergraduate and postgraduate education. The paradox is this: the things we find we have most thoroughly *learned* often turn out to have been the least systematically *taught*. Few of life's most important lessons are learned as the result of formal instruction – not language, not relationships, not (whatever our public schools may believe) how to behave at a party or in a shipwreck. Oh I know there are exceptions – reading, writing, arithmetic, the anatomy of the femoral triangle – but even in these cases no-one explicitly taught us how to *want* to learn these practical skills. And once we had learned the *wanting*, the details were just details.

In Vocational Training for General Practice, attempting as we are to stand eight years of hospital-orientated medical training on its head in only twelve short months, two over-reactions are sometimes seen. The first is *'over-teach'*, in which the unfortunate Trainee is desperately belaboured with curriculum, assessment and educational paradigm much as the heretics of old were excommunicated by bell, book and candle. The other is *'over-trust'*: to leave everything to chance, hoping that the Trainee will absorb what is needed by, and only by, the osmotic process of 'sitting with Nellie'. Both extremes take equally scant account of how real human beings really learn the things that really matter.

This issue – how real human beings really learn the things that really matter – is the subject of this chapter and the next. The preceding chapter proposed that effective education in the area of values, beliefs and motivation was 'the difference that makes the difference', and offered the hope that this need not be so daunting a task because the teacher has an under-recognised ally – the pupil's innate learning mechanisms whom I intend to christen the 'Inner Apprentice'. I want to begin this chapter by going right back to basics, asking what knowledge is, and how people come to modify their particular version of it. In so doing we shall be laying a conceptual framework for understanding and influencing motivation, values and beliefs which is substantially at odds with educational orthodoxy but not, I hope, with common sense and experience.

KNOWING AND LEARNING

> The Brain – is wider than the Sky –
> For – put them side by side –
> The one the other will contain
> With ease – and You – beside –
>
> The Brain is deeper than the sea –
> For – hold them – Blue to Blue –
> The one the other will absorb –
> As Sponges – Buckets – do –

(Emily Dickinson, c.1862)

As a working definition of learning, 'the acquisition of knowledge' will do. But the questions are begged; what do we mean by *knowledge*, and what's the point of our knowing things?

Despite all the aeons of mankind's evolutionary history, we remain frail bubbles in the universe's turmoil, parasites living on borrowed energy, our near-miraculous complexity battered by the tide of entropy that in time will engulf us. As we live out the 'meanwhile' of our individual existences, we each carry with us a store of knowledge which protects our identity from dissolution as an astronaut's life support system protects him from the lethal vacuum of space. If I were to attempt to clarify what 'knowledge' means by establishing its opposite, that antithesis would not be 'ignorance', nor the 'skills and attitudes' of the curriculum theorists, but instead something much more general – helplessness. Knowledge is the opposite of helplessness.

Consider simply what it means to *know* something. In everyday speech we say:

"I *know* the dose of penicillin";

"I *know* how to inject a tennis elbow";

90

"I *know* a fool when I see one";

"I *know* how you feel";

"I *know* that boy's not right for her";

"I *know* that my Redeemer liveth".

There are at least five domains wherein knowledge can be said to reside. We can know things:

— in our *heads* (the domain of factual knowledge);
— in our *muscles* (the domain of manual and technical accomplishment);
— in our *guts* (the domain of emotion, intuition and motivation);
— in our *hearts* (the domain of beliefs, values, moral and aesthetic judgements);
— in our *souls* (the domain of transcendent experience).

The common factor in all these domains is that knowledge consists of information put to good use. Knowledge is information that at one time was external to us and un-owned by us, but which we have subsequently encountered and selected, processed, incorporated and taken into ownership in such a way that (for the time being at least) it serves the function of helping us to understand and therefore control some aspect of our environment or experience. We encounter a fresh source of information, internalise some version of it, and allow it to modify our overall repertoire of thought and behaviour in ways which we hope will make the task of preserving physical and psychological integrity that bit easier. In a phrase:

> *Knowledge is information that works.*

We each have our own knowledge store, in a state of dynamic equilibrium between processes of accretion and depletion. On one hand are all the means at our disposal to increase knowledge: we can actively or passively acquire fresh information, or develop new ways of using old information. On the other hand are all the ways knowledge can decay. Synaptic networks undergo disuse atrophy, neurochemicals lose their fizz, and we forget. Old information finds itself overlaid or contradicted by new.

Our total behavioural repertoire – thoughts, feelings and actions – whose effectiveness the knowledge store exists to maintain, is also in a state of balance. Unless reliably updated as events unfold, habitual response patterns lose their adaptive usefulness and become an encumbrance. For us to acquire increased cognitive and behavioural options is generally helpful, enabling us to meet previously unmet needs, to survive in previously threatening circumstances, and to understand what was previously mysterious. However, some old responses lose their appropriateness and become liabilities. What we took for facts become time-expired; the habits and skills of a lifetime turn out to restrict the acquisition of more up-to-date versions; adherence to cherished beliefs and values may prove to have led us to paint ourselves into a corner. What we previously 'knew' no longer works, and we had best be shot of it.

It seems that we have been endowed by natural selection with learning processes that enable us – much of the time at least – to keep our knowledge store reasonably matched to the demands of our circumstances. Otherwise we shouldn't have survived as a species. By and large we learn what we need to learn when we need to learn it. We seem able to sense, albeit often subliminally, *when* fresh knowledge is needed and also *where* it is to be found.

This notion – that there is 'something inside us' able to tell what we need to learn and where to look for the means of learning it – is profound in its implications. It is at odds with the deep structure of most educational institutions, where the implied belief is that goal-directed learning is unlikely to occur in the absence of externally-imposed assessment and curriculum. But Socrates for one knew it to be true. In all his dialogues we can see him working to engage this 'something inside his listeners' where realisation might dawn. Socrates' style of questioning led his interlocutors to *aporia*, the crossroads of their beliefs. In this state of cognitive instability they found they not only had identified what it was they would need in order to relieve their discomfiture, but also realised they had arrived at exactly the point, intellectually and motivationally, where they were best placed to discover it. The medieval craft-masters, too, seem to have had an intuitive grasp of this principle in their conduct of apprenticeship. The apprentices found that each successive phase of their training, however formidable it might appear at the time, released in them the perception of what skill they next needed to acquire and the realisation that it did indeed lie within their reach. And I hope to show that a sound basis for both the theory and the practice of contemporary vocational education is this same principle:

> *People are intrinsically self-educating,*
> *as long as the right information is provided*
> *in the right way at the right time.*

THE INNER APPRENTICE

I have found it helpful to anthropomorphise these ideas. Let me introduce you to the Inner Apprentice. We shall be better teachers and learners if we get to know him and his ways.

The Inner Apprentice – mine's a 'he', though yours might not be – is the little person inside who organises our learning for us. His job is to make as sure as he can that we always have enough knowledge to meet our ever-changing informational needs. So moment by moment and year by year the Inner Apprentice diligently monitors our personal knowledge store. He can tell (usually, but not always) when our knowledge is working smoothly. And he can tell (usually, but not always) when it is not; and then he acts. The Inner Apprentice resembles the foreman in charge of a warehouse, who has an inventory of everything the warehouse is meant to contain and who is in charge of its through-put. He scans the shelves, stock-taking: "We're a bit short of facts over here – better get some more in; there's been a run on manual skills, and the suppliers are up-dating the specification; yes, we're OK in the emotions department; that last lot of values didn't fit too well and we had some complaints; the dust's getting a bit thick on that crate of old beliefs but we might as well hang on to them for the moment."

When the Inner Apprentice registers a knowledge gap or an ac-cumulation of out-of-date information that no longer works, he does something about it. Three things, in fact. The first is to draw our attention in a variety of ways to the fact that a knowledge need exists. Secondly, he scans the environment for learning opportunities and resources where the necessary information might be found and does his best to point them out, so that the new knowledge requirements can be satisfied. Thirdly, once learning has occurred and our information stores are working effectively again, he signals 'mission accomplished'.

Such is the three-phase response of an Inner Apprentice faced with a 'crisis learning need'. At other quieter times, when our knowledge is sufficient for our immediate needs and there's no rush job on, the Inner Apprentice is working to his own long-term agenda. Apprenticeships as we have seen have a trajectory to them, an optimum course over an extended time period during which short-term objectives succeed each other in a sequence or hierarchy leading towards fulfilment of the greater mission. Our 'inner apprenticeship' is no exception. In addition to short-term vicissitudes, there is a a universal trajectory to human learning which it is also the function of the Inner Apprentice to monitor. This 'trajectory of the inner apprenticeship' is what Maslow has described in his well-known hierarchy of human needs, to which we shall return in Part IV. First let me try to show you what I mean by the Inner Apprentice in action, telling us what we need to learn and knowing where to look for it. I'll take examples from several domains of knowledge.

The Inner Apprentice in action

In the domain of 'head knowledge', where facts are the currency, examples of inner-directed learning are two a penny. But even here a moment's introspection will confirm that the learning process is more complicated than simple educational theory portrays.

A patient consults me about a rash I don't immediately recognise: such dermatological information as I have in my knowledge store doesn't work on this occasion. I can tell I have a learning need from my feelings of puzzlement and helplessness, from the way I shift in my seat, avoid eye contact and start to talk medico-bluff, and from the way my thought processes try to coerce the appearances of this rash to fit a pattern I *would* recognise. All these cues, which subjectively I know only too well and some of which the astute patient will also spot, are signals from my Inner Apprentice. The Inner Apprentice will scan my predicament for the means of salvation. So I quickly find myself considering various options, either for accessing new information or making do with the old. For instance I might reach for a textbook, or go and get someone else's opinion, or make an outpatient referral, all of which would generate the necessary fresh information. If I didn't like to admit my ignorance, I could make an excuse to leave the room and consult a textbook out of sight of the patient, or say "Try this cream and come back in a week". Which option I choose will be governed by the relative weighting of the various conflicting values which are evoked by the particular circumstances. In this example, professional competence and professional pride are potentially at odds (unless I can reframe the skilful management of ignorance as a professional virtue). What I ultimately decide to do depends on whether my self-esteem is bolstered more by honesty or the illusion of infallibility. Whichever option I choose is likely to feel at the time to be the 'right' one, i.e. in accordance with my prevailing value system. My Inner Apprentice will then tell me that I have 'done the right thing' – I shall look, feel and behave satisfied, and shall think to myself that I 'know' how to handle a similar situation in future. Note that my new 'knowledge' may or may not be factually accurate. The Inner Apprentice may only have learned a new surreptitious way of making do with ignorance. But for the time being the knowledge store will again be functional, and the immediate challenge averted.

Note also that the generation and choice of learning strategies are mainly *unconscious* processes, not conscious ones. The realisation of ignorance usually takes us by surprise and is seldom the result of conscious analysis. When we wonder what to do about it we don't work systematically through algorithms and decision trees, however much some educators might like us to: more likely, we find ourselves being carried along by trains of thought whose route and destination we cannot fully control. Human learning is neither fully rational nor completely haphazard; rather, it is mediated by a mixture of conscious, preconscious and unconscious forces which will serve us better if we understand them better. Educational strategies need to be aligned with innate learning mechanisms, at as many psychological levels as possible. My excuse for coining the notion of an Inner Apprentice is wanting to invoke the depths of our potential for learning as well as the shallows, and also to convey a sense of their owner-friendliness.

Much of what takes place during higher professional training comes under the rubric of 'skills training', where 'head knowledge' has to be integrated into co-ordinated patterns of cognitive and manual dexterity. Some purely technical skills, such as injecting a tennis elbow or removing an ingrowing toe-nail, can be adequately learned in the way just described for the acquisition of factual knowledge. With relatively simple skills such as this, no different in principle from others already in the repertoire, the Inner Apprentice says in effect, "Just give me the facts, and then I'll know how to do the job." But many professional skills are of a higher order of complexity, calling not only for new information but also for new ways of processing that information, for new ways of perceiving, analysing and interpreting, and for the attributing of new significance to familiar material. This category includes the adaptation of the principles of clinical management and therapeutics to the specific setting of General Practice, as well as what are sometimes called 'people skills' – personnel management, team-work, and consultation skills. Attempts to teach these skills in the same instructional mode that we usually employ to impart facts often meet with disappointing results. In skills training, factual knowledge, though necessary at some stage, is neither prerequisite nor sufficient. Telling, or even showing, is not always the best way to help a pupil acquire complex skills. The Inner Apprentice is not a particularly good listener. His concentration wanders. While the rest of the class is reciting French irregular verbs he'd be that kid at the back with the faraway look, a copy of *Paris Match* under his desk, already in his mind's eye strolling on the left bank of the Seine or the beach at Saint Tropez . . . If you want to get the Inner Apprentice's attention, it's better to ask him questions.

A useful lesson in how the Inner Apprentice learns skills is to be found in an unexpected quarter – sports coaching. Let's say two people want to learn to hit a golf ball cleanly, sweetly and straight. They're complete novices. They take lessons from two professional coaches, both perfectly competent, but with different coaching styles. In fantasy, let's eavesdrop on their lessons.

The first novice golfer goes to a conventional coach. In his lesson he will probably be instructed in a number of key concepts about the golf swing – the grip, the stance, the address, the pivot, the follow-through. He will be told to keep his eye on the ball, his head still, his left arm straight, his shoulder pointing towards the ball. He must remember to pause at the top, to hit through the ball, to transfer the weight, to keep the clubhead square, to turn the hips (more than that, but not as much as *that!*), until his still head is reeling, his straight left arm turned to jelly, and his hips ready to turn and run. He is at risk of paralysis by over-instruction.

His friend goes to a coach of a different persuasion, one who understands how best to school the Inner Apprentice. Inspired by the work of Timothy Gallwey [1], the 'Inner Game' coach appreciates how too much instruction can get in the way of improvement by generating a distracting chatter of criticism and advice within the player's mind. This internal distraction can itself be distracted in turn, by having the player pay attention to certain external events and sensations which keep his mind focused in the here-and-now [2].

Observe the process of this alternative lesson. It might begin with the coach asking his pupil to "hit a few balls in whatever way seems natural to you". From the graceless contortions that follow it is clear that the pupil 'knows' that golf is an underarm game descended from certain forms of medieval combat. Undeterred, the coach resists the temptation to adopt the role of expert and instruct the pupil in technique. Instead he asks the pupil to set himself a concrete goal for today's lesson. The goal has to be:

– *realistic*, i.e. within the pupil's physical capabilities and achievable within the available time;

— *positively framed*, i.e. couched in terms of performance the pupil positively *does* want, rather than faults he does not;
— *specific* and *measurable*, i.e. something objective an external observer could assess as well as the pupil; and
— *deserving*, i.e. important and challenging enough to sustain the pupil's interest for the duration of the lesson.

"All I want is never to hit another slice ever again," is *not* a suitable goal. It's not realistic, it's negatively framed, it's not measurable (how straight has a ball got to fly before it doesn't count as a 'slice'?), and, since swopping the slice for a permanent hook would satisfy the goal as stated, it's not deserving enough.

Better would be, "By the end of the lesson, I want to hit a five-iron shot within 10 degrees either side of straight, with a lofted trajectory, 5 times out of 10." This mission statement satisfies the criteria, being *realistic* (attainable by a novice within an hour or two), *positively framed* (no mention here of hooks, slices, shanks and other gremlins best not named), *specific* and *measurable* (a theodolite and protractor could in theory settle any dispute), and *deserving* (as anyone who has ever experienced the ridiculous addictive and tantalising fascination of a single well-struck golf shot will know).

And now we can witness the uncanny potential of the Inner Apprentice, with a goal clearly envisioned, for sensing what learning process will bring that goal to fruition and where the necessary help and information are to be found. The Inner Apprentice sets to work, guiding the focus of attention of both pupil and coach, keeping his fingers crossed that they will trust him and not try to analyse or interfere too soon.

The golf lesson resumes with the pupil attempting a few more swings. Because he knows that lessons are supposed to be about improvement, and at this early stage the workings of the Inner Apprentice are still subliminal, the pupil will almost invariably follow each attempt with self-critical comments, progressing to requests for corrective instruction. "That was lousy. That was a bit more like it. That was nearly a good one. What did I do wrong that time? Am I holding the club right? You show me."

"For the moment," the 'Inner Game' coach replies, "it's enough for you just to observe, quite neutrally, the outcome of each swing. Don't evaluate: just notice. For now, tell me what you *see*, not what you *think*."

"OK. That one went along the ground, about 50 yards. That one was better – sorry, that one went over a hundred yards and would have cleared that tree easily, but it was twenty degrees off to the left."

And so on. Having achieved the beginnings of a shift in his pupil from 'judgemental mode' to 'awareness mode', the coach now intersperses a series of awareness-raising questions (ARQs) which have the effect, and *only* the effect, of focussing the pupil's attention onto here-and-now awareness of his body sensations. The pupil may already have some preconceptions about what it is that he *ought* to be paying attention to, but the awareness-centred coach will not collude with his pupil's intellect when it tries to take control of this early stage of the lesson. However random or unexpected or incongruous they may appear, those physical sensations and perceptions to which the pupil finds his attention being unwittingly drawn are in fact signals from his Inner Apprentice as to where moment-by-moment opportunities for effective learning and rapid improvement reside. Watch and listen.

> *Coach:* Stop for a moment. What sensations in your body have you become aware of during those last few swings?
>
> *Pupil:* I don't think I'm swinging my arms right.

(This is not a reply in the required terms of physical sensations. So the coach asks a further ARQ.)

> *Coach:* What have you noticed that makes you think that?
>
> *Pupil:* My arms don't feel right.
>
> *Coach:* 'Right' is what you *don't* feel. What is it you *do* feel?
>
> *Pupil:* Muscle tension.
>
> *Coach:* Whereabouts?
>
> *Pupil:* Errrm . . .
>
> *Coach:* If you're not sure, take a few more swings. Notice exactly where it is you feel the muscle tension, and then tell me.

The coach, having succeeded in identifying the sensory focus of his pupil's attention, is now concerned to elicit as much detail about it as the pupil's interest will sustain. The pupil swings a few more times. Imagine his state of mind as he does so. He has no idea whether the swing is 'right' or 'wrong'. All he knows is that some feeling in his arms is what has claimed his attention, and that for the time being he will trust the coach to make appropriate use of that information. In order to answer the question, "Whereabouts is the tension located?", his attention temporarily becomes fully focused on his arms to the exclusion of all other thoughts or sensations. For the time being, he has little concern if any for how the golf balls are flying. He is no longer 'best guessing' what he thinks is required of him: he has become awareness-centred rather than goal-, process- or outcome-centred. A few swings later he is in a position to reply.

> *Pupil:*   The tension's here, in my left upper arm mainly, on the inner side, about halfway between shoulder and elbow.

The coach, sensitively judging his language and timing, now develops his pupil's interest in this apparently arbitrary sensation with a series of ARQs which engage and maintain his full present-centred attention. 'What?', 'where?', 'when?, 'how?' and 'how much?' are questions which achieve this purpose. 'Why?' is not. 'Why?' questions tend to destroy present-centred awareness, and produce a flip into an analytic mode of response in which the pupil distances himself from his immediate sensory reality, and tends to justify the status quo instead of experimenting with new responses. ARQs suitable for this stage of the golf lesson might include:

- "*What* does the tension feel like? Describe it. "
- "*Where* exactly is it located? Is it only there, or somewhere else as well? Which is more or less?"
- "*When* do you feel this tension? All the time? Equally throughout the swing? When is it most? When least?"
- "*How* can you tell that what you're feeling is tension? How do you know whether it's increasing or decreasing?"
- "*How much* tension is there? A lot or a little? On a scale of 0 to 5, how much was there that time? How are you deciding that was a 3, and not a 2?"

And so on. The coach's task is to keep the ARQs coming as long as the pupil's absorption in the phenomenon of arm tension can be genuinely sustained. As long as there is curiosity present, he maximises it. If the pupil finds he can't answer a particular question, he hits a few more shots until his sensory awareness is keen enough to do so – or until he finds himself becoming more interested in something else.

The fascination of arm tension is of course limited. After a period of concentration on this, the pupil's attention will spontaneously shift, ARQs or no ARQs, to a new focus such as the sound of clubhead on ball, the inclination of the neck, or the varying pressure on the balls of the feet. The coach needs to spot this shift of attention when it occurs, either by periodically asking directly, or by recognising from tone of voice and minimal behavioural cues that the pupil's curiosity has become re-directed. He then asks ARQs couched to elicit full appreciation of the new focus.

So within a given span of inner-directed attention, its focus may vary. There is also a limit to the period for which inner-directed attention can be usefully sustained at all, regardless of focus. This period is usually a small number of minutes, after which a need to focus externally once more reasserts itself. When this happens, coach and pupil step back, straighten up, and then reflect and comment on what has been happening – what has been discovered, what is now being wondered, what might next be tried. The pupil's intellectual and analytical powers become important at this stage of the learning process if there is to be a sense of comprehension and ownership of whatever lessons are being learned. This is the stage where 'Why?' questions can be dealt with, advice given, demonstration and modelling offered. Before long, however, both pupil and coach feel ready once more to explore the inner sensorium through awareness-raising questions. In this way a rhythmic cycle of awareness-centred learning is established, in which there is a pendulum-like oscillation between internally- and externally-directed attention.

And what has been happening to performance during this carry-on? Surprise, surprise – more and more of the golf balls are sweetly struck and are flying straight and true! To his great delight the pupil notices how far he is already advancing towards his own self-imposed goal. He may not yet know quite how, but the evidence of his eyes is that without being told, he has learned. For those who equate learning with instruction and effort, the sensation of learning a skill by this method of coached explora-tion is an engaging novelty. Laughter, exhilaration and a renewal of energy are frequently experienced.

"That's all very well, but . . ."

The sporting example I have given of assisting the Inner Apprentice to acquire skills by the non-judgemental tracking of awareness is perhaps of no great cosmic consequence. Furthermore, I have couched my account in deliberately light-hearted terms, since my own personal experience has been that to be coached in this way is an enjoyable, intriguing and unlaboured process. Scepticism, however, is a natural and indeed necessary response at this point, if the potential contribution of aware-ness-centred methods to professional education is to be clarified and exploited. For I contend that in this process of skill acquisition by discovery rather than by instruction there can be discerned a powerful and universal learning methodology, supplementary and complementary to more traditional structures. Questions ought now to be arising in the reader's mind – questions which need to be answered if scepticism is to give way to curiosity and persuasion. Let us conduct a dialectic with an imaginary interlocutor.

"Are you kidding? Are you really saying that this gimmicky way of learning golf has anything of substance to contribute to the serious business of professional training?"

Certainly. There is a universal phenomenon operating here which is perhaps more easily discerned in a sporting setting, where the stakes are not too high and where we therefore dare risk questioning any assumption that the traditional ways of teaching are the only possible ones. If we divorce process from content, what am I saying? Simply that, when not unduly pressured, people can be assisted to set *themselves* goals which are realistic and timely, in the sense of being what they most need to learn at that particular time in their development. An externally-imposed curriculum is not always necessary. Furthermore, there is an intrinsic unconscious learning process at work which can not only sense *what* is ready to be learned but also indicate *how*. This unconscious process, which I call the Inner Apprentice, operates by guiding the awareness and attention of the learner towards those cues in the learning environment which, if attended to, will prove to be relevant and opportune. The Inner Apprentice is a shy and sensitive soul, easily intimidated by too much instruction, thriving best in an atmosphere of non-judgemental curiosity. The best way to coax it into co-operation is by means of awareness-raising techniques.

"So you say. What hard evidence do you have for all this?"

In the field of sports training evidence is copious. I first came across it in the work of Timothy Gallwey, the American erstwhile tennis coach and more recently consultant in training methods to a variety of industrial and corporate business enterprises. In his famous book *The Inner Game of Tennis*, published in 1974 [1], Gallwey showed convincingly how the chief obstacle to improving tennis skills is a distracting internal dialogue between a carping, criticising, bossy part of the mind (Self 1 in Gallwey's terminology) and a shyer, easily frightened but naturally talented part (Self 2) that could learn and perform perfectly well if only it wasn't nagged and bullied and ordered about and told what to try and do. Gallwey's solution was a range of coaching methods that distract Self 1, by giving it the task of non-judgementally perceiving here-and-now events such as the bounce of the ball or the instant of impact of ball on racquet. Gallwey subsequently generalised his 'Inner Game' methods to golf and skiing, with great success.

"How come your golf's still so lousy then?"

Ouch. Because awareness-centred coaching, though effective, isn't the whole story. There's also a need for follow-up, rehearsal and regular practice in order to consolidate, and that's where I fall down.

While researching this book I made the acquaintance of David Hemery, the hurdling gold-medallist in the 1968 Olympiad. Hemery's interests now are in raising the standards of British sports coaching. He and his associates are systematically training coaches in 'coaching by mental awareness', and the transcript of the 'Inner Golf' lesson is based on one of their sessions. This method of coaching has now been adopted in upwards of a dozen sports at national level. For me when I experienced this approach, it highlighted the fact that coaching skills are quite separate from performance skills (although some fortunate individuals possess both). It was possible, for instance, for novice coaches, including me, to assist Hemery in hurdles training through awareness-raising questioning that allowed him to follow the imperatives of his own attention as it ranged in turn over the point of heel contact on the ground, proprioceptive cues from the flexed knee and so on. Of these technicalities I have absolutely no knowledge, but facilitating the emergence of Hemery's awareness of them as he practised was clearly performance-enhancing for him. I found this humbling yet tremendously exciting. The challenge is to identify the key elements of awareness-centred coaching, and to see if they prove transferable to a wider set of skills than purely sporting ones. More specifically, I had the hunch that herein might lie an approach to training in professional values, beliefs and motivation – 'the difference that makes the difference' – areas where, as we have seen, the traditional educational paradigm is inappropriate.

"That remains to be seen. But why the 'Inner Apprentice'? In fact, why call awareness-based learning anything at all?"

Firstly, it's a phrase that lodges in the memory, and as a cue to recall that's important. But really it's a reminder that professional training is not a process of force-feeding with knowledge and skills. It also involves setting the said knowledge and skills in the context of a coherent set of values and beliefs, underpinned by a motivation towards excellence which, as we have seen, seems to have been the hallmark of effective apprenticeships in a variety of cultures. People's innate learning mechanisms are highly personal, highly sensitive and also, if allowed to be, highly reliable. Trainers don't have to flog their Trainees into action with lashings of curriculum and assessment. That's undignified and disrespectful. Moreover, since the medium is at odds with the stated message that professionals take responsibility for their own education, it's often ineffectual. I'd like the phrase 'Inner Apprentice' to lend academic respectability to such things as trust and dignity and individuality and respect, qualities which don't always seem to find a natural home within the traditional educational paradigm.

"So far what you've said about the Inner Apprentice has been an analogy, a metaphor for learning processes you claim exist. If I'm to take this analogy seriously, I need to be satisfied that there are corresponding processes explicable in neurological and biological terms as well as metaphorical."

And so you should. At some point the analogising has to correspond with physiological reality or else be ranked as fiction. Back to the golf lesson. An effective golf swing (i.e. one that reliably impels the ball in the intended trajectory) is a matter of balance, timing and muscular co-ordination. In general all these are under cerebellar and sub-cortical control dependent on feedback from afferent proprioceptive nerve impulses. In other words the body can tell by the way it feels whether or not muscles are co-ordinated, and agonists appropriately balanced with antagonists. Presumably there is also for the individual golfer a swing which will be his or her personal best approximation to the ideal. I think what must be happening is that, when the experimental swing departs significantly from this ideal, there arises some degree of muscle tension or sensory awareness which grabs the pupil's conscious attention. Inefficient muscle contraction causes tension or sensations which cross the threshold into conscious awareness. Conscious efforts to correct the source of this signal are largely ineffective, since muscle control at this level is not the domain of volition but of involuntary processes. What these involuntary control systems need in order to be effective is adequate and detailed proprioceptive feedback, enabling sub-cortical pathways to effect the necessary adjustments. This is what the awareness-raising questioning process provides. That's the best I can do with the 'golf' example. But it seems plausible to me.

"Even if that's all true for a golf swing, surely you can't assume that similar processes operate in the realms of cognitive and attitudinal learning, these factors that you say are the difference that makes the difference in professional training?"

You can't assume it, certainly, but it's a reasonable and testable hypothesis. After all, nature seems generally to use Occam's razor, the labour-saving principle that similar needs in different contexts are more efficiently served by variations on a single theme than by radically different ones.

Anyway, let's reflect upon the question of whether the Inner Apprentice can learn concepts, values and insights in this non-directive and awareness-centred way. Isn't the whole edifice of psychotherapy based on this foundation? Say what you like about Freud, the central premise of psychoanalysis has survived a century of mixed hagiology and scorn. That premise is that people signal their deepest needs, truest feelings and most urgent priorities not in clear and unambiguous language, but indirectly and subliminally – in free association, fantasies and dreams, jokes and slips of the tongue. When the patient climbs onto the analyst's couch, it's in these ways that his or her Inner Apprentice brings the psychotherapeutic agenda for that particular occasion into conscious awareness. Some part of the patient's mind 'knows', or at any rate 'signals', where the educative attention of analyst and analysand is most profitably to be directed that day. The ability to pick up these signals is arguably at least as important a therapeutic factor as whatever interpretation the analyst's training places upon them. Subsequent generations of psychologists have added to the list of cues we now recognise as signalling the possibility of therapeutic change: behavioural rituals, body language, facial expression, tone of voice, metaphors, speech hesitancies, omissions, ambiguities and circumlocutions, and so on. Psychotherapy can be thought of as the establishment of a learning environment in which, largely by means of awareness-raising questions, these tentative signals from the Inner Apprentice are coaxed by non-judgemental attention into a clarity from which important lessons can be safely learned.

In all client-centred therapies there is a rhythm of communication between client and therapist, gradually building the intensity of their joint attention. The client offers whatever thought has currently come to the forefront of his or her mind; the therapist then heightens and develops that thought, assisting in the exploration of its ramifications until it acquires the power of transformational insight. In every school of counselling the role of counsellor is that of midwife to an answer that already lies within. Advice, the "If I were you" solution, is of less value by virtue of being second-hand. The same conclusion, self-discovered, is more enduringly mutative (change-producing).

In their astonishingly astute and evocative book *Mutative Metaphors in Psychotherapy: The Aeolian Mode* [3], Murray Cox and Alice Theilgaard quote some remarks of a psychotherapy patient who was aware of how the paying of high-quality attention can evince awareness of the appropriate starting point for learning [op. cit. pp. 48–9]. "You don't begin at the surface", she wrote, "not because you begin at the depth, but because *you* don't begin. You induce beginning in me. . . The closer we get to something that is out of *both* our depths, the more at home I feel and the more I actually feel *I know more than you about everything, including me.* It could be that I put it in your mind because I know the springboard I need. *I know which door I want you to open on my behalf.*"

Viola, an old American cleaning lady, put it rather more raunchily. She had borrowed her employer's copy of *Lady Chatterley's Lover*, D. H. Lawrence's story of the unfulfilled gentlewoman and the randy game-keeper. It was returned with this note: "Thanks! Missus Chatterley didn't know what she *wanted*, but she sure'n hell knew what she *needed!*" [4].

That 'I' that knows which door it wants opened on my behalf is the Inner Apprentice. It's self-educating, as long as the right information is provided in the right way at the right time. Now Vocational Training is of course neither sport nor therapy – probably it's quite a lot of both! – but since we can discern similar principles of coaching at work in such apparently unrelated fields, let's see what might ensue if we allow awareness-centred teaching to challenge the monopoly of the traditional educational paradigm.

"I can't believe you're saying there's no place for formal and systematic teaching in post-graduate medical training."

Indeed not. Curriculum, syllabus, formal tuition, assessment both for-mative and summative – these are the interlocking components of a highly structured educational tradition with much to be proud of. And, in fact, as we've seen in the examples of sport and psychotherapy, awareness-centred coaching is itself a no less highly structured method of teaching. It's just that the two structures are intended to bring about different effects. Curriculum-based teaching techniques are intended primarily to guide the actions of the teacher. Awareness-centred teaching is structured primarily to guide the experience of the learner. Neither invalidates the other. The outcome of each is necessary. Neither is sufficient. Each should be used for what it's best at.

"Actually it seems to me, when you pare away this talk of an Inner Apprentice, all you're saying is that there are some things people can work out for themselves, given time, using trial and error."

I'm certainly saying that, but not *just* that. . .

"I mean, you've given that list of 14 hallmarks of excellence which I'll concede are not best served by traditionally-organised teaching. And you're clearly going to claim that awareness-centred teaching is more successful in the areas you consider to be vital, namely beliefs, values and motivation. On the other hand, I'm sure you'll admit that a lot of medicine – not just the facts and figures, but a lot of the skills as well – simply

doesn't *consist of knowledge that by any stretch of the imagination can be said to be pre-resident within the pupil, like a sleeping Princess needing nothing more than the kiss of a Prince Charming in order to awaken. Slashing away at a golf ball while you ask yourself how your arm feels is all very well, but I wouldn't want to be the patient of someone who was learning medicine that way."*

Nor I. At least, I wouldn't want to be the patient of someone who was learning therapeutics or joint injection techniques in so experimental a way. Equally, though, I wouldn't want to be the patient of a Trainee who hadn't yet learned to be tolerant of his patients' shortcomings, or to acknowledge his own, simply because his Trainer didn't know how to foster those values. Nor of one who only asked open questions when being videoed; nor one who was only planning on reading the journals until the MRCGP Orals were safely out of the way!

I *am* saying that the scope and array of what people can learn through awareness-raising techniques is wider and at the same time more far-reaching that we have previously credited. I *am* suggesting that aware-ness-raising techniques can succeed in fostering higher-order attributes, such as motivation and values, where didactic curriculum-based teaching fails. I *am* saying that the educational circumstances in which people can best learn through awareness-raising do lie within the control of a teacher who can foster and optimize them. And I *am* saying that there are professionally important qualities which, like the insights resulting from psychotherapy, can only be self-discovered in the presence of a mentor skilled enough to pilot the student's self-awareness through a sea of irrelevances and distractions.

Let's think for a moment about the role of a formal curriculum in Vocational Training. Will you bear with another analogy – the curriculum as menu?

My favourite restaurant has a menu that changes only very gradually. Over the course of a year or so, I visit it often enough to have tried most of the dishes on the *à la carte* menu. Having seen the totality of what is available, I make my own choices as to what to eat on any given visit. Each choice is the resultant of various forces, including my personal likes and dislikes, my curiosity, other meals I may have had recently, and my sense of trust that the chef is unlikely to present a dish unworthy of the establishment's reputation. If the restaurant only offered a set *table d'hôte* menu, I shouldn't enjoy going so much, because eventually I should come to feel resentful at the lack of choice and suspicious that the chef's abilities couldn't match the aspirations of his customers. And if the waiter was too pushy in his recommendations I should opt for something different just to assert my individuality. The role of a curriculum should be that of an *à la carte* menu – to define a decision-space which both enlarges the choices of the customers and enables them to do justice to whatever powers of appreciation they possess. An over-assertive curriculum reduces a Traineeship to education's equivalent of dinner at Fawlty Towers. But a sensitively-used curriculum can serve to spread before a Trainee a tempting catalogue of possibilities which his professional predecessors have found valuable. It's a question of who assigns priorities to this array, and of whose choice is to be trusted. Traditionally the curriculum, through its agent the Trainer, assumes these responsibilities. I'm suggesting that the pupil's Inner Apprentice can be trusted to make informed judgements no less reliably. Curriculum should be used to open up an area of potential growth; the Inner Apprentice, if allowed to, will ensure that the Trainee expands into it, because that is its nature.

A further benefit of enabling the pupil to discover his own 'inner curriculum' and establish his own learning priorities is that whatever choices he makes will be endowed with a greater motivational energy than is the case with an externally-imposed syllabus, no matter how subtle the imposition. The curriculum is of course more familiar to the coach than to the pupil, but that does not diminish the value of enabling the pupil to chart his own course through it. If that process of charting was left to the pupil's *conscious* preferences, prone as they are to self-deception and inertia, I should be more worried. But if, through familiarity with the Inner Apprentice and its ways, we as teachers can come to recognise our pupils' *unconscious* learning needs as they are constantly being signalled to us, we need not be quite so fearful of a Trainee-led trajectory.

"So you're suggesting that when Trainer and Trainee are planning their teaching, mere discussion isn't enough . . ."

No, because if you simply ask people what they think they need to learn, the answer will come in the form of consciously selected words; and we know that words are often less reliable indicators of people's true needs and feelings than their non-verbal communications. I'm advocating greater attention to, and reliance on, non-verbal indications of an inner curriculum.

". . . and instead the day-by-day educational programme should be guided by the various topics and concerns to which the Trainee finds attention being unconsciously drawn."

Day-by-day and also moment-by moment, yes – in the same way that a compass needle, in the absence of intrusive magnetic fields, can be trusted to align itself at all times towards the pole. The pull of the learner's attention, like the pull of the Earth's magnetic field, is no less reliable for being invisible.

To put it another way:

> *What matters, gets noticed;*
> *what gets noticed, matters.*

"Apart from that story of the golf lesson, which is interesting but not necessarily an exact parallel, you haven't said anything about the way these educational needs are signalled non-verbally, nor about how they can be used to help a Trainee learn."

No, not yet. That's what we'll come on to in the next chapter.

"If for the time being I allow that a Trainee's ever-changing interests and awareness might eventually lead him through all the curricular territory he's capable of exploring, isn't there nevertheless a place for a Trainer to offer short-cuts. What's wrong with a bit of guidance, a bit of old-fashioned didactic telling? Why deny a Trainee the chance of profiting from someone else's experience, by saying, 'Look – try this. I think now would be a good time to look at so-and-so. Let me suggest something.'?"

There's nothing intrinsically *wrong* with didactic teaching – except the assumption that it is intrinsically *right!* It's terribly easy and tempting for a teacher to assume that, because *he* understands something of unquestionable importance, the best and most efficient way to have a pupil reach the same understanding is to tell him, loud, clear and forcefully. The didactic approach leaves out one very important factor – timing: is the pupil ready to learn that particular lesson? Is it the lesson he's at that moment most hungry for? And is formal instruction the best way of having him learn it, or might exploration of his own awareness not prove more valuable?

Rhythmicity

The question of getting a balance between instruction-based and awareness-based learning is vital, because it connects with what has already been said about the 'trajectory' of educational programmes. The trajectory of any learning episode emerges from the interplay of, and oscillation between, two distinct mental 'sets' which we saw in the golf example and will doubtless recognise from the ways we ourselves have learned in the past.

Human conscious awareness is a creature possessing dual nationality, with a passport to travel freely between each of two homelands. One is the realm beyond our skin, the realm of things and places and events and other people. This is the so-called 'objective' domain, which we infer from the constant sampling activity of our sensory systems and accept as real since everybody else seems to. The other is the internal subjective realm of our own thoughts and feelings, a private and invisible world of which we are the sole inhabitant. At any given moment, it seems, we can be aware of either one, or (more commonly) we can be partly aware of both simultaneously.

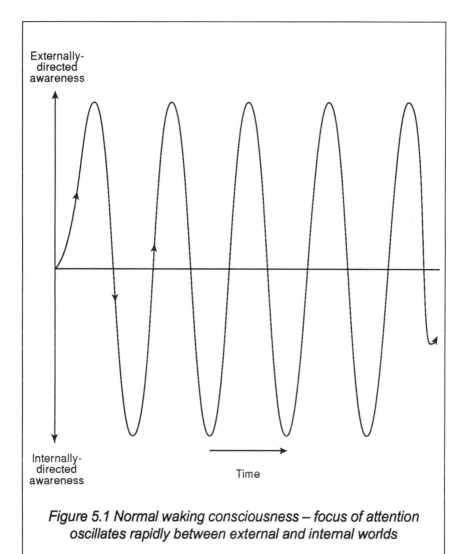

Externally-directed awareness

Internally-directed awareness

Time

Figure 5.1 Normal waking consciousness – focus of attention oscillates rapidly between external and internal worlds

On closer inspection, what passes for normal waking consciousness can be seen to consist of rapid alternations in which of these two worlds – external or internal – forms the immediate focus for our attention (see Figure 5.1). As we react moment by moment, aware of everything in general and nothing in particular, our attention is flicking rapidly back and forth every few seconds, now inwardly and now outwardly directed. Something 'catches our eye', some event registers in the outside world, and attention locks onto it. An instant later some thought occurs, some sensation arises, and quite automatically our attention switches for the moment to become inner-directed. I say 'automatically': all this means is that the mechanisms whereby attention is directed are located at preconscious or unconscious levels. Such a form of psychological autopilot is clearly necessary if human consciousness is ever to cope with the virtual infinity of information endlessly clamouring for a response.

Most of the time this inwards/outwards alternation, this shuttling of attention back and forth between objective and subjective domains, takes place so fast and so subliminally that we scarcely notice it. But under certain circumstances the attention's rate of oscillation can be slowed down and brought under more conscious control. When this happens, and the autopilot is disengaged, there is time for us to attend more selectively and more thoughtfully to what we are doing. There is time to recognise more of what is going on inside us, time to scan the environment more thoroughly for the threats and opportunities it contains, time to plan what we say and do in response. When the attention is reined in, harnessed and controlled, we cease to be merely reactive and instead become proactive, taking charge of events, thinking things through, reviewing our performance, making choices, creating fresh options – in a nutshell, dealing optimally with new information; in a word, learning (see Figure 5.2) A state of mind in which the wayward attention is brought under conscious control and appropriately focussed seems to provide the most favourable circumstances for learning to occur.

This 'psychological autopilot', the 'black box' that decides what we become aware of and what we attend to, is the Inner Apprentice we all possess. The setting up, maintenance and educational use of conditions of controlled attention constitutes the 'awareness-centred learning' for which this book is a plea.

In awareness-centred learning there is an educational alliance between, on the one hand, the learner's Inner Apprentice, recognising and signalling the existence of learning needs, and on the other the teacher's ability to slow down, intensify and guide the learner's focus of attention. The golf lesson was one example of this process in action; a psychotherapy

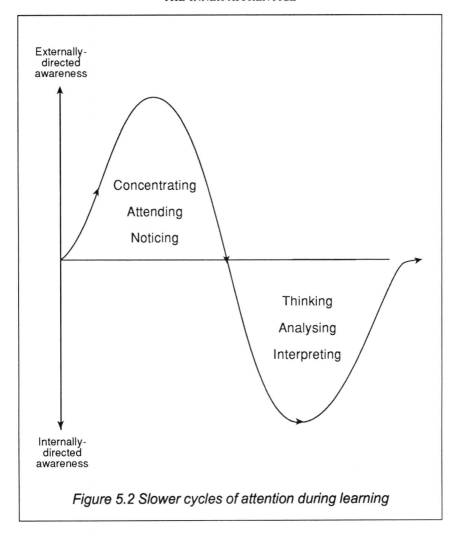

Figure 5.2 Slower cycles of attention during learning

session is another. (I make no apology for portraying psychotherapy as a form of education: 'teaching' in my present context is a process not of instruction but of cue-recognition and awareness-raising.) The teacher sets up conditions of controlled attention in which all the cues the learner becomes aware of can be explored as fully as possible. This awareness-raising phase alternates with episodes of consolidation. What has been discovered through heightened awareness needs to be evaluated, taken on board and integrated with what was known or believed previously. The moment-by-moment trajectory of each episode of learning is a dance to this alternating rhythm. Figure 5.3 illustrates this.

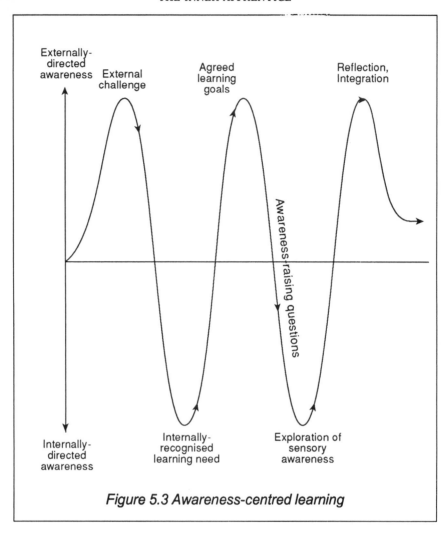

Figure 5.3 Awareness-centred learning

The same processes also contribute to the emergence of a longer-term trajectory. We have already seen examples – historical and fictional in Chapters 1 and 2, professional and contemporary in Chapter 3 – of how apprentices in various settings embark Icarus-like on their own particular trajectories. Within the safety of the relationship of tutelage the novice is encouraged first to envision a state of mastery which endows the apprenticeship with a motivating sense of mission. During the ensuing weeks and months, learning episodes occur whose overall resultant is an expansion of the apprentice's capabilities and self-awareness. These are interspersed with periods of review, when the results of previous learning are incorporated into the repertoire. Performance is raised to a higher level, affording the journeyman a vision of yet further territory to be explored

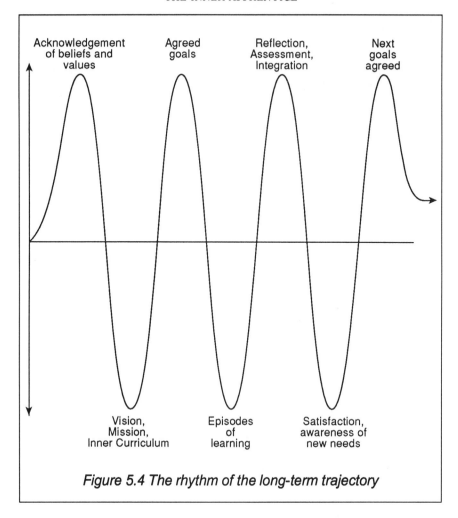

Figure 5.4 The rhythm of the long-term trajectory

and yet higher goals to be aspired to (see Figure 5.4). In Part IV we shall see how sequential self-selected goals of the inner curriculum are hierarchically arranged. As one succeeds another and is in its turn superseded by something more sophisticated, a trajectory of attainment is created.

There seems thus to be an underlying unity of process linking the ebb and flow of everyday awareness with the attainment of our secret dreams. The same dynamic – attention in, attention out; in, out – seems to be operating on all the educational timescales, moment-by-moment, month-by-month.

SUMMARY

A person's knowledge store is, to a greater extent than traditional educational methods often acknowledge, self-maintaining. An innate learning mechanism, largely preconscious and unconscious and here christened the Inner Apprentice:

(1) Registers and indicates when a need arises for new learning to take place;

(2) Establishes and prioritises the individual's inner curriculum of personally-relevant learning goals;

(3) Is able to identify and locate potentially mutative information in the environment; and

(4) (If the conditions are right) makes appropriate use of self-selected educational opportunities.

The Inner Apprentice learns best from cycles of non-judgemental awareness-raising alternating with periods of review, reflection, discussion and consolidation.

The Inner Apprentice communicates (1) by unconsciously adjusting perceptual mechanisms and (2) by controlling the focus of conscious attention. From a learning point of view, what matters gets noticed; and what gets noticed, matters.

From the wide range of settings in which these learning processes can be identified, it seems possible that some of the most important professional attributes, including values and beliefs, might be learned in similar awareness-centred ways.

An awareness-centred approach to teaching and learning requires a teacher to suppress his own curricular agenda in favour of the curriculum generated by the learner's Inner Apprentice. For this process to be reliable and effective, skill is needed in recognising cues indicative of an Inner Curriculum, combined with the ability to respond with the right information presented to the learner in the right way and at the right time.

To assist in the fostering of such skills is the ambition of the remainder of this book. General principles will be advanced in the next chapter. Part IV, 'Teaching The Inner Apprentice', includes a selection of practical strategies and techniques.

Chapter 6
How the Inner Apprentice learns

Education does not consist merely in adorning the memory and
enlightening the understanding.
Its main business should be to direct the will.

Joubert, 1842

In this chapter we shall explore the general principles of coaching the
Inner Apprentice. My aim is to set the stage for detailed consideration of
modifications teachers might make to their usual teaching strategies if
they want their efforts to be in closest alignment with their students' in-
built learning mechanisms. Human beings, so the axiom goes, appear to
be intrinsically self-educating, as long as the right information is presented
to them in the right way at the right time. What *is* the 'right' information?
How can we tell what's *right* in this context? What *is* the 'right' way to
present educational information? When *is* the 'right' time; and again,
how can we tell?

Figure 6.1 summarises in graphic form the sequential process whereby the
Inner Apprentice does its learning. If this book has a nutshell, Figure 6.1
is it. Some of the terms are unfamiliar; nonetheless I believe the ideas they
refer to will be immediately recognisable, especially to teachers. After all,
at some point in our lives we have all had the experience of being well
taught, and at some point we have all been able to make a significant
contribution to the learning and development of someone else. It is with
these intrinsic and universal learning and teaching abilities that I'm
hoping to establish contact. The way you'll be able to tell whether or not
I'm succeeding will be by registering periodical little frissons of recognition as I attempt to render conscious and systematic an array of
perceptions that may perhaps previously have been subconscious and
unstructured. If your own Inner Apprentice occasionally mutters "Oh
that; yes, I know *that*!", we'll be on the same wavelength.

Unfamiliar circumstances generate
a need for MUTATIVE INFORMATION.
This need results in a disquieting state of
COGNITIVE DISSONANCE,
which is felt subjectively, and which is also
indicated by behavioural MINIMAL CUES
detectable by an attuned and perceptive teacher.
At the pivotal POINT OF KAIROS,
the learner's Inner Apprentice
attempts to reduce cognitive dissonance,
either
by discounting the mutative information,
or,
(helped by AWARENESS–RAISING QUESTIONING,
and under conditions of SAFE INSECURITY)
by restructuring the knowledge store,
including its beliefs and values,
i.e learning.
Repertoire–enhancing learning
produces a sense of
COGNITIVE RESONANCE,
and in extreme cases, a powerful EPIPHANY,
which also have learner–specific minimal cues.
The legacy of cognitive resonance is
an educational EXPANSION SPACE,
hierarchically organised,
into which the learner grows and develops
as the TRAJECTORY OF APPRENTICESHIP unfolds.

Figure 6.1 How the Inner Apprentice learns

In this chapter I'll begin with some definitions of the terms I'm using. Then I'll expand on them somewhat, suggesting how the various elements come together into an understanding of the way intrinsic learning mechanisms operate to keep our knowledge store in the best possible shape. The key concept is an unsettling feeling called 'cognitive dissonance' – a 'pain in the self-image' – that indicates the need to learn. From this I hope it will become clear that effective teaching strategies begin at the 'micro' level, where the priority needs of a learner's Inner Curriculum are signalled by minimal verbal and non-verbal cues.

DEFINITIONS

'Mutative information'

(as in 'trans*mute*', '*mut*ation') – information capable of producing lasting and valuable change. The term '*mutative*' describes information capable of significantly augmenting and restructuring the knowledge store after fresh circumstances have revealed important competence-threatening shortcomings. For example, to an Edinburgh resident, a street map of London may be merely interesting. To someone lost in London's West End, the same information would be truly mutative.

'Cognitive dissonance'

– a term coined in 1957 by Festinger, whose 'theory of cognitive dissonance' described how people always tend, retrospectively, to justify their own decisions and behaviours [1,2]. Cognitive dissonance (CD) is the unsettling feeling of mental tension experienced when confronted with the evidence of one's own inadequacy. Cognitive dissonance is a disquieting state, which we feel compelled to resolve and which therefore generates a potential energy for learning.

'Minimal cues'

– the physical signs of mental states. Evidence of private thoughts and feelings leaks out in the form of micro-behavioural cues which other people can detect. Minimal cues can be verbal and non-verbal. Verbal cues may be 'linguistic', i.e. a person's choice of words and figures of speech; or 'paralinguistic', i.e. the pace, pitch, volume, rhythm and tonal range of the voice. Non-verbal cues include posture, gesture, muscle tone, breathing patterns, direction of gaze, eye contact, and facial expression. Intuition and 'reading between the lines' stem from our ability to interpret minimal cues.

'Point of kairos'

– a pivotal point of maximal opportunity during an educational episode, where, depending on whether or not mutative information is available, significant learning either does or does not take place. '*Kairos*' in Greek means the right time for action, the critical moment, an auspicious period when conditions and portents are at their most favourable. By analogy, at an educational point of kairos the learner can most clearly recognise the nub of the issue, the heart of the problem, and is most receptive to mutative information. In Chapter 1 we eavesdropped on Socrates as he taught, his questions leading an interlocutor on until he confronted the limits of his own thought in a state of helpless '*aporia*'. This is an example, a particularly uncomfortable one, of a point of kairos. At such a time, cognitive dissonance is at its most intense and the potential for restructuring the knowledge store correspondingly greatest.

A single tutorial session may contain one or more points of kairos, of different magnitudes and in different domains of knowledge.

'Awareness-raising questioning'

– a style of enquiry designed to elicit as fully and non-judgementally as possible a person's immediately available state of knowledge, thoughts, perceptions, beliefs and values, without attempting to criticise or modify them.

'Safe insecurity'

– a 'just tolerable' state of cognitive dissonance, when a pupil is aware of a learning need and feels accordingly vulnerable, but is at the same time sufficiently trusting of the context to resist any tendency to defensive re-entrenchment. Safety and insecurity are optimally balanced. Without some degree of insecurity there would be no motivation to learn; while without safety there would be no progress.

'Cognitive resonance'

– a term of my own coinage, to describe the converse of cognitive dissonance. Cognitive resonance is the positive feeling we get after cognitive dissonance has been resolved and successful learning has taken place. When mutative information has had the desired effect and the knowledge store is restored to equilibrium, there is a release of mental tension experienced as satisfaction, insight or understanding. Like cognitive dissonance, cognitive resonance has its own minimal cues – tell-tale linguistic, paralinguistic and behavioural signs.

'Epiphany'

– an unusually powerful feeling of cognitive resonance when a particularly far-reaching or deep-going piece of learning has taken place. Lessons of 'epiphany' proportions are few and far between, but are intensely felt at the time and are long remembered. As 'the scales fall from our eyes', there may be strong attendant emotions such as relief, elation, insight or humility.

'Expansion space'

– the area of educational 'unexplored territory' representing the goals and interests next on the learner's Inner Curriculum. An analogy would be the environmental and chemical gradients that determine the direction of an amoeba's extending pseudopodium, behind which the organism as a whole will follow. Successful completion of one piece of learning releases a readiness for the next. An educational expansion space cannot be arbitrarily imposed, although a skilled teacher may assist in clarifying it.

'Trajectory of apprenticeship'

– the sequence of expansion spaces successfully opened up as an extended educational programme unfolds. The series of expansion spaces is not effectively dictated by an imposed curriculum. Rather, it follows an intrinsic developmental sequence of priorities, hierarchically arranged, in that readiness for one depends on successful attainment of those immediately preceding.

AN OVERALL VIEW

It would be helpful if, having grappled with these definitions and explanations, you would now have a second look at the 'nutshell' summary of how the Inner Apprentice learns (Figure 6.1, page 116). I hope it makes a little more sense now.

If I were to attempt a diagnosis of why programmes of postgraduate professional education sometimes underachieve, it would be along the following lines. There has been over-reliance on a simplistic view of adult learning, based on arrays of curriculum-derived objectives and on insensitive tools of formal assessment. Conventional teaching methods have neglected (and sometimes come into abrasive collision with) the full potential of students' intrinsic learning mechanisms. By increasing their awareness of the power and scope of the Inner Apprentice's contribution, teachers might more efficiently ensure that their own energy to teach and their pupils' energy to learn are brought into better alignment and synchronisation.

A teacher who is 'inner-orientated' is constantly trying to spot, by tracking minimal cues, what it is, and when and how, the pupil is ready to learn next. The learning agenda, on all timescales, is the pupil's *own* compromise between two factors: the knowledge deficits that come to the pupil's attention in the course of daily experience; and his or her current beliefs and values, and whatever sense of mission flows from them. Both factors are amenable to mutative awareness-raising questioning.

The learner's own Inner Curriculum, as signalled by the spontaneously changing focus of attention and by the ebb and flow of cognitive dissonance, is a more powerful and reliable educational ally than we may have realised. Trainers with a 'difficult' Trainee are often heard lamenting, "You can lead a horse to water but you can't make him drink". In fact, the Inner Apprentice is a horse perennially thirsty; it's just that he knows better than the stable-hand where the water is freshest, and that it isn't necessarily to be found in the communal drinking-trough of a pre-ordained curriculum.

If you think about the various circumstances in which learning needs make themselves felt, *unfamiliarity* seems to be the common factor. For a Vocational Trainee undergoing in-service training 'on the job', unfamiliarity can strike from many different directions. First, the daily round of unpredictable clinical work mercilessly highlights the shortfall between existing and required knowledge. It seems likely that a twelve-month period in general practice is long enough for all important professional challenges to be encountered at some point, at least in representative form. Secondly, most Trainers like to anticipate the inevitable by conducting set-piece tutorials on topics they expect Trainees to be unfamiliar with. Thirdly, the check-lists and rating scales in common use bombard their readers with unfamiliar items (though with how much motivational impact is debatable). Fourthly, circumstances may call for professional beliefs and values alien to the Trainee's own current ones and in that sense unfamiliar. Finally, Trainees themselves actively pursue aspects of the unfamiliar that intrigue them as part of a self-imposed career mission.

No-one enjoys the awareness of personal fallibility; and to register a learning need, however helpful in the long run, is to acknowledge that right now we'd be better if we were different. The complex reactions we feel in response to such a discovery are called cognitive dissonance. Cognitive dissonance comes in various flavours, all of them to some extent unsettling, and the fact that it's unsettling shows in minimal cues, some of which have already been mentioned. Too intense an experience of cognitive dissonance causes us to withdraw into our shell, like a startled tortoise. But lesser degrees of CD can be capitalised upon. An inner-orientated teacher can recognise the signs of cognitive dissonance signalling a learning opportunity, and can contrive to maintain it at a tolerable level of safe insecurity. By recognising the points of kairos when readiness to learn is at its strongest, and by then combining awareness-raising questioning and judiciously presented mutative information in the alternating rhythm described at the end of Chapter 5, the teacher can sustain an optimal learning environment until cognitive dissonance is abated. The complementary state of cognitive resonance – the sense that once again all's right with one's internal world – then replaces it, signalling restitution of the knowledge store.

It often seems to happen that the learning needs arising in a given time-span seem thematically linked, and coalesce for days or weeks at a time within one particular domain of knowledge. For example, at the start of a Traineeship the Trainee's priority needs are largely to learn the practice's working arrangements, and the names and roles of its staff. Soon a need asserts itself for basic general practice 'survival skills' like managing the common minor illnesses and knowing what forms to fill in. Later on the Trainee develops a readiness to learn about more sophisticated aspects of practice, such as consulting skills, or family dynamics, or finance. Familiarisation with each small parcel of knowledge seems to open up an expansion space into which the Trainee's interest will next be drawn. Successive expansion spaces follow a hierarchy of priorities, imposing its own inherent sequence and structure on the trajectory of a Traineeship. In animal ethology there is the concept of 'sensitive periods' – windows of opportunity when certain behaviours can be learned, which do not open ahead of their due time and close remorselessly if the chance is missed. The same seems to hold true of human apprenticeships, though perhaps less deterministically.

COGNITIVE HOMEOSTASIS:
MAINTAINING AN EFFECTIVE KNOWLEDGE STORE

Staying well-informed is an essential biological process, like staying well-nourished. So let's recall some basic biology. When studying physiology we were introduced to Claude Bernard's principle of the 'milieu intérieur', the inner environment of physical and biochemical parameters needing to be maintained within certain ranges for essential living processes to function effectively. Vital systems are controlled and regulated by the feedback mechanism of *homeostasis*. The body has some means of sensing when a given variable begins to stray beyond the limits of its effective range; the cues that signal this impending instability then initiate compensatory processes, reversing the errant trend; finally, when normality is restored, a second feedback message signals the end of the need to compensate.

Examples genetic, biochemical and metabolic of this homeostatic process are numerous and well understood in medical contexts. Many homeostatically-regulated processes take place at molecular and cellular levels, such as the array of hormonal feedback mechanisms involving hypothalamus, pituitary and endocrine glands. We remain unconscious of most of our metabolic homeostasis, at least until it begins to fail. Other more sophisticated homeostatic processes, particularly those where complex behaviour is part of the corrective mechanism, impinge also on conscious awareness. For example: control of blood sugar resides at the molecular level with insulin, adrenalin and their friends. But this unconscious process has its conscious correlates. Falling blood sugar is signalled consciously as the sensation of hunger, which prompts the food-seeking behaviour necessary for its relief. In turn, once the meal is under way, the feeling of fullness signals when it is time to stop.

Human learning is governed by analogous homeostatic processes. Look again at Figure 6.1 (How the Inner Apprentice learns, p.116): you will discern in it the essential features of a homeostatic system. In this case the 'variable' needing to be maintained within an effective range is the knowledge store, which has to be kept in a fit state to ensure psychological and biological survival in a constantly changing environment. The sense of cognitive dissonance (CD) arises as a signal when unfamiliar or challenging circumstances reveal an impending inadequacy in the knowledge store. CD is felt as a sense of threat to our self-image, and is the conscious indication of the need for change. CD instigates the search for, and incorporation of, mutative information which will restore adequate knowledge. Cognitive resonance (CR) is the signal indicating when we

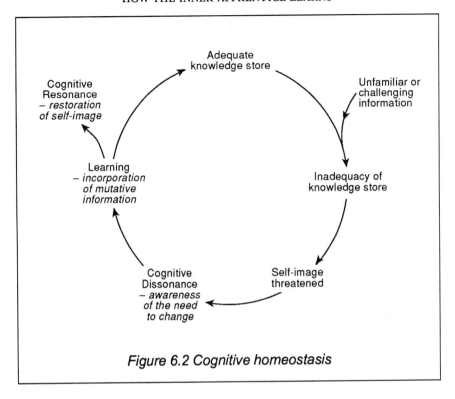

Figure 6.2 Cognitive homeostasis

once again have knowledge sufficient for our requirements. CR is felt subjectively as a return of the self-image's sense of well-being (see Figure 6.2, 'Cognitive homeostasis').

The self-image

In order to understand more clearly how CD and CR act as indicators of the learning process, we need to consider the notion of a 'self-image'. For CD and CR are, respectively, the feelings of mounting unease and restored confidence in the image we have of ourselves.

We all have an image of the sort of person we are: in fact, we have *several* self-images. There is the private image of the person we deep down believe ourselves to be – usually a saintly paragon with a few, very few, endearing warts. There are also the various public faces we like to present to other people. We are very protective of our self-images. Indeed we have to be, since we spend every waking moment in the company of one or other of them. Anything that undermines or contradicts the way we like to think of ourselves is potentially disruptive to our sense of personal worth, and this we find worrying. A jeopardised self-image, when either we ourselves or those whose opinions matter to us think badly of the way we are coming across, produces extremely bothersome and unsettling sensations. The term 'cognitive dissonance' refers to the various disturbing feelings we experience when our self-image has been hurt – when the person we are revealed to be falls short in our own estimation of the person we had liked to think we were. Because the experience of CD implies that we are failing to match up to requirements, we are strongly motivated to reduce it. When some personal inadequacy is revealed, particularly if the evidence is public and undeniable, CD results in our taking steps (consciously or unconsciously) to limit the damage to the self-image and to restore self-esteem. It does this by causing us to think various defensive thoughts, experience various defensive sensations, and behave in various defensive ways.

When experience conflicts with self-image, one or the other has to give way. 'Facts' are not sacrosanct to the human psyche. A favourite way of dispelling CD is to re-interpret the events that produced it, so that they can be perceived in a light more favourable to us and more in keeping with the principles and beliefs we thought we held dear. Evidence of our own inadequacy can be denied, contradicted and distorted, its origin discounted, and any threat to the self-image thereby sidestepped. Nietzsche beautifully described this human penchant for donning rose-tinted spectacles before looking in mirrors: *'"I have done that," says my memory. "I cannot have done that" – says my pride, and remains adamant. At last – memory yields.'* Some examples may make this clearer.

Late for surgery and driving in a hurry, I overtake injudiciously and am hooted by another motorist: believing myself to be a good driver, I tell myself there was really bags of room, and thereby convert guilt into righteous indignation. A patient describes at length bizarre and inconsistent symptoms: believing myself to be a kind and sensitive doctor, I rationalise my irritation with the thought that some people are enough to try the patience of a saint; if I don't give of my best it just goes to show that verbal diarrhoea carries a morbidity. The consultation looks like overrunning by fifteen minutes: I justify the unnecessary blood test that terminates it by reminding myself how important it is not to miss physical disease. The next patient's rash defeats me: believing myself 'good at skins', I diagnose 'atypical eczema' and recommend a trial of antibiotic-containing steroid cream. Detected in this catch-penny ruse by my Trainee, I convert my embarrassment into an opportunity to expatiate upon the merits in General Practice of diagnosis by hypothesis-testing and on the therapeutic use of time. And so on. In fairness, these distortions of facts to fit psychological needs are seldom done with conscious calculating intent to deceive. But the process of preserving the self-image by a shift of perception is the same defence mechanism that leads in extremity to paranoia.

Another way of reducing cognitive dissonance is to allow the self-image itself to undergo change, albeit painfully. When events take us down a peg, one way to adjust is to 'stop kidding ourselves', amputating the area of gangrenous self-esteem, and settling for the knowledge that we are after all flawed and ignoble mortals, no better than we ought to be. CD handled this way has the potential to lead us towards insight, humility and self-knowledge; all laudable ends, no doubt, but not without their dangers also. Taking the previous paragraph's saga as an example: I needn't be a road-hog, but self-confessed timidity that will not overtake even a milk-float is itself a hazard to those behind me in the queue. If I resolve to allow every discursive consultation to run its uninterrupted course, the results of my martyrdom to patient-centredness may be to rob some patients of necessary boundaries, to keep others waiting intolerably, and give myself an ulcer. The dermatologist won't thank me for referring every doubtful rash; and if to prescribe Betnovate-N means being black-balled from training . . . well! CD-reduction by denial may be a paranoid trait, but trying to achieve the same result by relentless whittling away of the self-image carries a risk of depression as its end-point.

Fine descriptions of these two polarised ways of dispelling CD – arrogant self-delusion on one hand and grovelling self-abasement on the other – are to be found in novels by E. M. Forster. The first is from *Howards End*. Helen Schlegel has been retrieved, amid scenes of confusion, by her aunt Mrs Munt from an unsuitable whirlwind romance with Paul Wilcox.

> Helen and her aunt returned to Wickham Place in a state of collapse, and for a little time Margaret *(Helen's sister)* had three invalids on her hands. Mrs Munt soon recovered. She possessed to a remarkable degree the power of distorting the past, and before many days were over she had forgotten the part played by her own imprudence in the catastrophe. Even at the crisis she had cried, "Thank goodness, poor Margaret is saved this!" which during the journey to London evolved into "It had to be gone through by someone," which in its turn ripened into the permanent form of "The one time I really did help Emily's girls was over the Wilcox business." But Helen was a more serious patient. New ideas had burst upon her like a thunderclap, and by them and by their reverberations she had been stunned. [3]

The second is from *A Passage To India*. Adela Quested, an emancipated young English girl visiting India for the first time, has accepted the local Doctor Aziz' socially daring invitation to a picnic at the Marabar caves. Miss Quested asks him,

> in her honest, decent, inquisitive way: "Have you one wife or more than one?"
>
> The question shocked the young man very much. It challenged a new conviction of his community, and new convictions are more sensitive than old. If she had said, "Do you worship one god or several?" he would not have objected. But to ask an educated Indian Moslem how many wives he has – appalling, hideous! He was in trouble how to conceal his confusion. "One, one in my own particular case," he spluttered, and let go of her hand. Quite a number of caves were at the top of the track, and thinking, "Damn the English even at their best," he plunged into one of them to recover his balance . . . He waited in his cave a minute, and lit a cigarette so that he could remark on rejoining her, "I bolted in to get out of the draught," or something of the sort. When he returned he found the guide alone . . . [4]

And because Aziz needed a few moments of solitude away from his guest to compose his affronted self-esteem, there occurred the unfortunate incident that was to prove his undoing.

CD as learning opportunity

Between these two extreme ways of resolving cognitive dissonance there is a third possibility. Cognitive dissonance can be resolved by *learning*. As we have seen, the function of cognitive homeostasis is to preserve the integrity of the self-image amidst daily psychological and environmental vicissitudes. CD arises whenever our knowledge store is challenged by circumstance and found wanting. In other words, CD is an indication of the immediate need to learn: the presence of CD is what defines the existence of a learning opportunity. CD tells the individual who experiences it (and also an attendant teacher with eyes and ears open to detect it) that now, *right now*, is a time when the Inner Apprentice has identified a gap in the knowledge store, and is motivated to remedy it. For remedy it it will, one way or another. If suitable mutative information is available, so well and good; growth-enhancing learning will take place. In the absence of acceptable and relevant information, however, the self-image's integrity will be restored by one or other of the two ultimately unfulfilling methods so well described by Forster. Had Mrs Munt been in therapy, or had Dr Aziz taken a course in assertiveness training, each might have emerged from Gethsemane a nobler character. But no source of mutative information was to hand; and so their windows of opportunity slammed shut. For only these three options exist – self-delusion, self-devaluation, or learning. As teachers, we have the clear duty to time and pace our interventions skilfully, so as to render the 'learning option' most likely.

Little pieces of cognitive homeostasis are going on all the time, many times each day. Faced with never-ending challenge and novelty, sometimes momentous but usually of no great significance, the Inner Apprentice is constantly making adjustments to the ways we think, perceive and behave. Most of these adjustments occur automatically and subliminally, so that we may not always recognise them for the episodes of learning they in fact are. We tend to reserve the term 'learning' for episodes of knowledge-acquisition on the grand scale, such as occur in formal lessons or as the result of a carefully engineered assessment process. But most human learning occurs in much smaller increments. Most human learning (and I believe the learning that ultimately makes the difference) is a process of creeping evolution – evolution not only in the domains of facts and skills but also, as we saw in Chapter 5, in the values and beliefs we cherish and in the sense of mission that motivates us.

And so it behoves teachers, as the paid facilitators of other people's learning, to develop competence not only in the 'set piece' teaching techniques based on curriculum and assessment, but also in the dynamics of 'micro-teaching' on a moment-by-moment timescale. When it comes to teaching the Inner Apprentice,

'Macro' may be macho, but 'micro' makes the difference.

MICRO-TEACHING

The natural home of 'inner-orientated' teaching is informal one-to-one tuition: topic tutorials, random case analyses, 'hot topic' case discussions and video consultation review. These are all occasions where the attention paid to the learner's knowledge gaps can be intense yet at the same time supportive. I like the phrase 'safe insecurity' as a description of these conditions where the learner's own Inner Curriculum can most readily be discerned and addressed.

I believe 'macro'-teaching based on curriculum-derived objectives and formal assessment is often inappropriate, inhibiting and insensitive in the context of one-to-one teaching. I mean 'insensitive' in both its meanings. 'Macro'-teaching, while it may satisfy some Trainer Selection Committees, can be insensitive to the paradoxical mix of vulnerability and sophistication exhibited by adult learners. Adult sensibilities are easily bruised by rigid teaching methods that cynical 14-year-olds manage to shrug off. 'Macro'-teaching is also insensitive in the sense of being too gross an approach where what needs to be learned resides principally in the domains of insights and values. It is like doing brain surgery with a machete. To concentrate on inner-directed teaching at so immediate and parochial a level is not, however, to abrogate responsibility to the greater curriculum. On the contrary; I shall hope to convince the reader that inner-directed teaching leads more naturally and comprehensively into the overall trajectory of professional education than does the conventional version. Inner-directed teaching and learning flourish in an atmosphere of safe insecurity. Too slavish an adherence to the doctrine of 'define/teach/assess' risks creating a spurious insecurity, poorly aligned with the learner's truly current learning needs. Furthermore, however hard a compassionate teacher may try to establish a safe feel to the formal assessment process, the inhibiting rigidity of the iron fist is inescapably detected within the proffered velvet glove. I believe that teaching to the Inner Curriculum is no less rigorous and comprehensive than its formal counterpart, and is capable of being more sensitively fine-tuned to the ever-changing priorities of the individual learner.

The minutiae of cognitive dissonance

Inner-directed teaching stands or falls on the ability to spot the physical signs of cognitive dissonance. An ability to recognise CD as it arises in a student is perhaps the single most valuable skill an inner-orientated teacher can develop. During everyday encounters with patients, and in such everyday educational settings as case discussion, video analysis and simple clinical gossip, the knowledge store is being actively and continuously accessed. All the time the Trainee's Inner Apprentice is performing its monitoring function. Its signals consist of constantly flickering hints of CD hovering on the margin of conscious awareness. While 'business as usual' is being transacted, we experience (if we learn to recognise it) a counterpoint of fluctuations in the nature and intensity of the accompanying emotional 'edge', signalling the coming and going of moments of educational opportunity.

Insecurity, nervousness
Fidgeting, restlessness
Self–consciousness, awkwardness, barrassment
Hesitancy, evasiveness
Guardedness, defensiveness
Aggression, hostility, brusqueness, irritation
Vocal and/or physical tension
'Avoidance' behaviour – reduced eye contact, physical backing–off
Day–dreaming, loss of concentration
Surprise, curiosity
Inappropriate humour or laughter
Sudden increase or decrease in energy level
Unexpected rush of emotion

Figure 6.3 Some 'symptoms' of Cognitive Dissonance,
indicating learning opportunities

The account and examples of CD so far presented may have implied that the jolts it causes to the self-image, and the consequent sense of instability, are substantial ones. And so it may be: in its most intense forms CD is powerfully manifest as guilt, shame, confusion, outrage, despair or mortification. But these are the large tremors on the human Richter scale, the primary colours on the emotional palette. Usually CD is encountered in less intense examples. We are here talking frissons and pastel shades. Figure 6.3 gives a list of some of its 'symptoms' – the ways that educationally-relevant CD may be experienced.

Part IV of this book, 'Teaching the Inner Apprentice', first goes into detail about how cognitive dissonance signalling an immediate learning need can be recognised by its minimal cues. There then follow chapters indicating how the information thus gleaned forms a basis for teaching strategies on all timescales.

Part IV
Teaching the
Inner Apprentice

I only wanted to set free
those who would enjoy teaching like this.

Elizabeth Irvine
(Lydia Rapoport lectures, 1974)

Chapter 7
Minimal cues

MINIMAL CUES – TELL-TALE SIGNS OF THE INNER CURRICULUM

A poem by Emily Dickinson begins as follows:

> There's a certain Slant of light,
> Winter Afternoons –
> That oppresses, like the Heft
> Of Cathedral Tunes –
> Heavenly Hurt, it gives us –
> We can find no scar,
> But internal difference,
> Where the Meanings are –

[1]

The teacher's job is to *detect* that certain 'slant of light' as it flickers in a pupil's face and eyes; to *hear* the resonances of 'cathedral tunes' in a pupil's voice; to *empathise* with the 'heavenly hurt' of cognitive dissonance; and to *sense*, long before scar formation can occur, the all-important tell-tale signs of 'internal difference where the meanings are'.

Cognitive dissonance – the herald of a learning opportunity – has symptoms, as summarized in Figure 6.3 (p.129). It also has tell-tale physical signs which it is the teacher's business to learn to recognise. The signs may vary from person to person, but there is enough uniformity to warrant some general descriptions. Individual variations between one pupil and another are quickly learned 'on the job' by the inner-directed teacher willing to appreciate their significance.

> *Minimal cues are the physical signs of mental states.*

I like the term 'minimal cues' to describe all the verbal and non-verbal signals we constantly emit as involuntary accompaniments to our private thoughts and feelings. To the discerning observer, minimal cues provide more reliable evidence of our true state of mind than the carefully-structured language behind which we tend to shelter. We often learn less from what people say than from what they *don't* say, or from how they look and sound while they're saying it. When on the look-out for clues as to what a pupil is ready to learn, a teacher 'listens with the eyes and watches with the ears'. The pupil's own account of what he or she needs to know is of course important, and must always be addressed. But without simultaneous attention being paid to the Inner Curriculum, largely unconsciously driven and non-verbally expressed, satisfaction of the pupil's arguably deeper and more radical educational needs is imperilled.

How is a teacher to discover this Inner Curriculum? By developing a heightened awareness of particular minimal cues. By listening not only to what's said but at the same time wondering, "What's *not* being said? What's *nearly* being said?; what *could* have been said but wasn't?; what's being glossed over or skirted around? What doesn't quite make sense? *How* is what's said being said?; how is it being expressed? What looks and sounds as if it *matters*?"

Educationally-relevant minimal cues are of three types. (The distinction may prove helpful when it comes to training oneself to spot them.) The first category is 'linguistic' cues, where the nuances of the exact choice of words are significant. Second are the 'para-linguistic' cues, where information is conveyed by the inflexion of the voice rather than the literal sense of the words. Finally, there are the 'non-verbal' cues of body language and facial expression.

LINGUISTIC CUES

Gambits and curtain-raisers

In my previous book on the consultation process [2], I suggested that the opening few moments of each consultation are particularly informative about the patient's agenda on that occasion. In order not to miss high-grade information communicated by the patient, a doctor does well to concentrate full attention on the patient's opening words, endeavouring to remain, initially at least, maximally receptive and minimally intrusive. I distinguished between two types of information contained in the patient's first remarks: an opening 'gambit', premeditated and often rehearsed, being the way the patient has consciously decided to express his or her reason for coming; and a 'curtain-raiser' – spontaneous and unrehearsed remarks, often trivial but sometimes revelatory, made immediately on entering the room and before presenting the intended gambit. Gambits indicate to the doctor a starting point where the patient feels secure, and from which the initial business of the consultation can be negotiated. Curtain-raisers are more indicative of the patient's mood, emotional state, values, beliefs and hidden agenda – all factors needing to be recognised by the doctor if underlying as well as superficial needs are to be met.

An example: a doctor concentrating exclusively on the opening gambit *"I've been getting a pain in my stomach"* is likely to hasten off down the medical track via history and examination in search of an organic diagnosis. This response may well be necessary; yet – in General Practice, where a basis in pathology for every presenting symptom cannot be universally assumed – it may also be insufficient. Consider what important clues are disclosed in the following impromptu curtain-raisers, and how much more sensitively and productively the consultation might flow if the doctor perceived them:

"I don't suppose it's anything serious, but . . ."
"You'll be getting fed up with me. Anyway, . . ."
(Deep sigh) "Errmmm . . ."
"It's probably just nerves, but . . ."
"Don't be giving me any of your pills . . ."
"I tried to get an appointment four days ago! Anyway . . ."
"Of course I usually see one of the other doctors . . ."

Not for the first time let us notice here an isomorphism between the clinical relationship of doctor to patient and the educational one of Trainer to Trainee. In many tutorial settings, especially random case discussions, a Trainee begins by offering a condensed account of a consultation. Such an opening gambit is often phrased in such a way as to attract the Trainer's attention to selected aspects of the case, where the Trainee perceives the need for help but at the same time wants that help to prove only minimally threatening to his or her self-image. A safe educational agenda is initially mooted. However, the safe and obvious agenda is not always the necessary one. If discussion is confined to consciously-identified topics, the risks exist of collusiveness, of developing blind-spots, and of postponing the appreciation of deeper layers and more complex issues. Since all human beings dislike cognitive dissonance, defensiveness is natural in students; no teacher should renege on the duty to handle their vulnerabilities gently and sensitively. Yet, as in the clinical example of the painful stomach, teaching that is necessary may not be sufficient. Teachers have a duty also to find safe ways of eliciting their pupils' more far-reaching educational needs. Within our present context, this means learning to recognise and interpret signals from the Inner Apprentice. The educational equivalent of the curtain-raiser is one such signal. The words Trainees use to introduce their descriptions of their own clinical work often contain 'leaked' signals of educational needs which have already been noted by the Inner Apprentice, even though the speaker is not as yet fully aware of their import.

Another example, this time educational: a Trainee describing a consultation with four-year-old Michael might offer as an opening gambit, "He was a child with otitis media: I gave him an antibiotic." This gambit effectively restricts the Trainer's response to asking whether the diagnosis was reliable, whether an antibiotic was necessary, and if so, which one. Thus constrained, discussion is likely to be brief, factual and relatively unenlightening to both parties. The Trainee sounds sure of the diagnosis, confident in the decision to prescribe, but willing to allow debate on the choice of antibiotic – a legitimate but unstretching issue. An even more deadly stymie would have been the gambit, "This was just a child with obvious otitis media: I prescribed ampicillin 125 mg qds for five days, to cover the possibility of a *Haemophilus* infection." (Next case, please.)

Consider, though, the wealth of minimal cues to an Inner Curriculum detectable in such curtain-raiser comments as:

"Oh yes, he was just a quickie . . ."
"I'd spent ages with the previous patient who was tired all the time . . ."
"Surgery was running late, but luckily . . ."
"At least there was *one* straightforward case . . ."
"*You* usually seem to see this child . . ."
"I think *everybody* must have seen this child . . ."
"I'd got the wrong child's notes at first . . ."
"I'd seen the sister last week with a cold . . ."
(Wry smile) "Oh yes, Michael! . . ."
"Oh yes, came with his father . . ."

Off-the-cuff scene-setting remarks like these can form the base for an educational safari into unexplored educational territory far lusher than might have been anticipated. The examples given could lead, for instance, into discussion of:

– time management;
– the 'tired all the time' patient;
– surgery appointment systems;
– the Trainee's expectations of General Practice workload;

- job stress;
- continuity of care;
- Balint's ideas on the 'collusion of anonymity';
- problems of reception staff;
- the management of minor illness;
- family dynamics;
- patients' health beliefs;
- awareness of the doctor's own feelings;
- or even the role of the Health Visitor!

Significant curtain-raisers indicate some degree of cognitive dissonance. In them can be heard the whispering, if not the clamouring, voice of the Inner Apprentice. Whatever gambit is consciously selected, recognition of associated learning needs at an unconscious level has already occurred, and leaks into unguarded speech in the form of a curtain-raiser. Let me, however, anticipate a question of emphasis which may worry the reader as we raise awareness of minimal cues. I am *not* suggesting that the obvious and straightforward should always yield to the covert and the complicated. I am *not* suggesting that every minimal cue to deep-going educational needs is immediately to be pounced upon and worried to death. For a Trainer always to be hunting to extinction every last nuance of every uttered word is at best inhibiting to a Trainee, and at worst irritating beyond measure. Educational hunches, like clinical ones, can be stored up until the moment is right to declare them. But the cues need to be noticed; for what is not noticed can *never* be addressed. The noticing *is* necessary, and, for the time being, sufficient.

Speech censoring

If you listen carefully to the flow of another person's speech it is possible to detect, within the overall sense that it conveys, moment-by-moment and word-by-word variations in the precision of the language used. Much of the time, 'what you hear is what is meant', with no room for misunderstanding. But at other times the speaker uses words and phrases that are to some extent vague, ambiguous, incomplete, circumlocutory, imprecise, non-specific. In other words you have to listen between the lines, make assumptions about the missing detail, and 'best guess' the speaker's true intended meaning. You get the feeling that some figures of speech and turns of phrase withhold at least as much information as they impart. So a graph of 'explicitness' against time would show a series of peaks and troughs. The inversion of this graph would chart the amount of work the listener would have to do in the form of supplementary questioning in order to retrieve the speaker's full meaning from the incomplete version.

Take for example the sentence, *"I told Jill the other day in no uncertain terms just what I thought."* Consider each of its component ideas, and notice how explicitly or otherwise they are expressed (Figure 7.1).

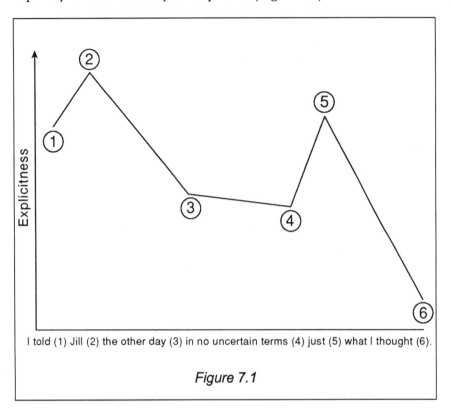

I told (1) Jill (2) the other day (3) in no uncertain terms (4) just (5) what I thought (6).

Figure 7.1

"I told" is fairly explicit; the only uncertainty is whether the telling was face-to-face, by phone, or by letter. The identity of *"Jill"* is bound to be unambiguous in the context of the conversation. *"The other day"* is moderately vague. We assume it refers to the recent past, probably within the last week, but if someone's alibi depended on it no jury would convict on this evidence. *"In no uncertain terms"* is interesting. We are to believe that what was said was brutally frank, but we can only guess at how it was expressed. The speaker may have sworn like a trooper, been icily sarcastic, barked like a barrack-room lawyer; or, for all we know, may have flannelled and soft-soaped, but wants us to think the opposite: we can't tell. *"Just"* probably means the same as *"no uncertain terms"*. But, depending on the emphasis and tone of voice, it might mean that the speaker *could* have discussed other matters, but chose not to; or that the speaker could have given the views of other people, but again chose not to. With *"what I thought"*, the imagination of the listener has to work

overtime. The phrase assumes that the speaker's views are known already, but in the context it is unlikely that in fact they are. If the listener also has strong views on the subject, he or she may assume that they are the same as the speaker's, a dangerous assumption. The sentence as a whole steers an erratic course between, on one hand, the comprehensiveness of "*I phoned Jill Smith at 11 a.m. the day before yesterday and told her that in my view she should divorce the swine immediately*", and on the other the colloquial but uninformative, "*Ooh I didn't half tell her!*"

In such a mixture of explicitness and ambiguity, detail and blurring, most of our conversational exchanges are conducted with a 'good enough' degree of mutual comprehension. But when the context is an educational one, it behoves us to pay a little more attention to these linguistic imprecisions. What's going on (we should wonder) when complete information *could* have been forthcoming but for some reason is withheld or concealed under a camouflage of imprecise phraseology? Usually it is not the result of deliberate intent to mislead. There are several possibly innocent reasons: humour; habit; a desire to tease or to prompt response; poverty of vocabulary; pressure of time; overlapping of the assumptive worlds of speaker and listener. Language fully detailed, free from all ambiguity, the language of the technical manual, unequivocal and unleavened with metaphor or whimsy, can be paralysingly dull. But the teacher's attuned ear, while not eschewing the conventions of normal conversation, should strain to detect those occasions when it has to guess, to make assumptions, to listen between the lines. For often language's smaller vaguenesses belie an unconscious attempt by the Inner Apprentice to protect the self-image from having its inadequacies exposed. In the example given, the speaker may not wish to reveal just how angry or abusive he or she could be, or how opinionated. If the image usually presented to the listener is softly-spoken and level-headed, such revelations may prove undermining. But as we know, in the right context a challenge to the self-image also creates an educational opportunity.

It's as if there was in our head a 'speech censor' whose job it is to monitor what we are about to say just before we say it. If the censor realises that we are about to say something that might show us in a bad light, or reveal some ignorance or shortcoming we should prefer to pass unnoticed, it modifies our choice of words, reducing the amount of hard and attributable information in what we say. In the resulting linguistic fog the self-image can usually slip away unwounded. The listener will be too preoccupied with having to 'fill in the gaps' to notice deficiencies in knowledge, memory or belief.

Looked at another way, however, speech censoring indicates a pre-conscious awareness of a learning need, and is therefore an educationally relevant phenomenon. Speech censoring is a coded signal from an Inner Apprentice that can foresee an incipient knowledge gap and can anticipate the associated cognitive dissonance, but isn't yet sure that suitably safe mutative information is at hand. In the *"I told Jill . . ."* example, at (3), (4) and (6) where the lack of explicit detail indicates speech censoring, the speaker's Inner Apprentice is signalling, *"I don't know whether it matters to you which day Jill and I spoke (3), whether you realise quite how forcefully I can express myself (4), or whether you'll approve of my opinion (6)."* Speech censoring represents the Inner Apprentice raising its head cautiously above the parapet to see whether it is amongst friends or foes: if the former, learning is possible; if the latter, it can retreat into the status quo.

Speech censoring reveals itself in various forms, any or all of which may alert a teacher to the presence of cognitive dissonance and thus indicate (if the teacher judges the moment to be right) a possible learning opportunity.

Omissions

Important specific details are left out, so that the listener has to ask supplementary questions. E.g. *"I prescribed an antibiotic"*. Which antibiotic? What dose? *"I'll get onto the social workers."* Why? And say what? The type and degree of the speaker's cognitive dissonance can be estimated from the type of supplementary the listener feels inclined to ask, and, more significantly, from whatever slight emotional charge – curiosity, irritation, humour – the listener feels in response to the omission.

Distortions

Essentially neutral events are described in such a way as to endow them with a meaning and significance they may not on the evidence possess. E.g. *"The patient demanded an antibiotic for his sore throat, so I did a little health education."* It is unlikely that the patient did anything as forceful as *demand*, or that the doctor's reply qualified as bona fide *health education*! Distortions often take the form of "I am right, you are misinformed, he is pig-ignorant". With this type of language, the speech censor forestalls criticism by implying that responsibility for any difficulties lies not with the speaker. When the self-image is defended by distortion, misrepresentations and misinterpretations may result.

Generalisations

The existence of a general and invariable rule, principle or property is implied, in order to disguise the lack of appropriate specific detail. E.g. *"I always check the blood pressure."* (But did you on *this* occasion?) *"I don't believe in high fibre diets."* (You don't believe *what* about them?) *"I've never understood skins."* (Really? Never anything at all?) *"We discused all the risk factors, and so on."* (Confess now: what did you say about what?) The speaker hopes that the listener will credit him with a sophistication not in fact possessed.

Hesitations and prevarications

Hesitations in the flow of speech are the footfalls of an Inner Apprentice treading cautiously amidst what it knows to be a minefield. Phrases like *"Errm. . .", "Well. . .", "I suppose. . ."*, or *"How shall I say?"* are all forms of speech censoring, buying time for the speaker to call up reserves of knowledge. The fluency and specificity of the next remark may indicate whether such reserves in fact exist.

Non sequiturs

One form of speech censoring often thought endearing or humorous is the everyday version of the schizophrenic's 'knight's move' speech. In an account of some sequence of events one or more intermediate steps, possibly wobbly ones, are left out or glossed over. For example, a Trainee who knows the side-effects of aspirin-like drugs but doesn't know how to inject a frozen shoulder may utter the non sequitur, *"I saw he'd had a duodenal ulcer, so I referred him for physiotherapy"*. (But duodenal ulcers aren't treated with physiotherapy!) A "Hold on a minute!" reaction is the listener's guide to spotting this form of speech censorship. Careful retrieval of the missing steps will reveal any significant knowledge gaps.

In ordinary conversation, speech censoring seldom needs to be challenged. "I know what *you* mean, and you know what *I* mean" is a good enough working assumption. But in a teaching and learning context, conversations are defined as potentially more than ordinary. To this end a teacher needs the ability to reserve a part of his or her attention for noticing these soft signals from the Inner Apprentice, and for judging the likelihood that they indicate a learning need worth addressing. Often a brief clarifying question or informative interruption is enough. Every now and then, however, such a convulsion of speech censoring occurs that the listening teacher can only think *"Wow!"* and switch into full awareness-raising mode. See how many forms of speech censoring you can identify in the following tutorial excerpt:

"Whenever they come in and come out with Tired All The Time you think, well, well I do at any rate – marital! By then of course I'd got hours behind, and no one had said. So anyway, I got a blood test . . ."

Value-laden phrases

As we saw in the first of the passages by E. M. Forster quoted in the previous chapter, one way of reducing the discomfiture of cognitive dissonance is to reinterpret the facts. When facts and self-image collide, almost without thinking we coerce our interpretation of the evidence into a version that bothers us less; we are thus spared the embarrassment of having to learn from painful experience.

Why is the need so strong in us always to be *right*? Why should it be so unsettling to discover that some things about ourselves could do with changing? Over millenia of human social evolution some Darwinian process seems to have favoured the cultural survival of the self-assured. What existential peril, what sabre-toothed tiger of the psyche lurks, against which self-justification is our best defence? Think on: for fossil evidence of our primordial egocentricity abounds in almost every breath of speech.

My theme is that cognitive dissonance matters: it hurts, minimal cues reveal it, but it can be learnt from. The CD induced when a gap shows up in our store of factual and practical knowledge is an acute distress, hot like a sprain or needing a rub like a stubbed toe. But dissonance in the domain of personal values, where self-esteem resides, is an altogether more prostrating affair, gnawing like a cancer, throbbing and festering like an abscess. In the section on speech censoring we saw how the Inner Apprentice cautiously explores the linguistic territory immediately ahead, lest an unguarded tongue betray a weakness. But if it is our value systems that are threatened, speech censoring is too passive a response. When values are at stake the Inner Apprentice prefers to take the offensive and get its retaliation in first. Our words come out fighting, bearing the colours and favours of the values they champion. Our choice of words asserts the way we need to see things if we are to live comfortably with them. We obey the righteous imperative; in phrases approving and pejorative by turns, in the nuances and niceties of emotive vocabulary, we proclaim, "Where it really counts, *I'm right!*" Think how many variations you have heard on the theme of "I have an enquiring mind, you are inquisitive, he is a nosey-parker."

Once you attune your ear, it will surprise you how much of everyday speech carries personal advertising in the form of value-laden phrases. English having such a large formal and colloquial vocabulary, we select from the available synonyms those whose associated values best coincide with our own. From people's choice of phrase we infer their beliefs, their priorities, their ethics and their feelings. We can tell (or think we can) what they esteem and what they deplore; what they support and what they oppose; what they think is right and important, and what wrong or inconsequential.

Eavesdrop on the value-laden language of doctors talking about patients. One patient *"goes on about"* a problem; whereas another is said to *"unburden"*. One *"asks for help with"* a symptom; another *"complains"* of it. Someone *"pesters"* the doctor about *"osteo-whatsits and chiro-thingies"*; but someone more congenial *"shows an interest in complementary medicine"*. One wife is *"concerned"* about her husband's drinking; another *"suffers from anxiety"* over it; while a third *"gets herself into a right state"*. She says her man is *"always legging it off down the boozer"*; but *he* can't see much harm in *"popping out for a quick jar with the lads."*

It is the hint of underlying value-systems that infuses humanity into conversation and spices it with individual opinion. Value-free emotionally-neutral descriptions of human affairs soon pall; moreover, the listener quickly suspects that less than the complete truth is being told. It is normal, therefore, that dialectic between teacher and learner should be conducted in uninhibited language naturally rich in value overtones. Yet, the setting being defined as an educational one, a teacher under-serves a pupil if too many value-rich cues are discounted as mere idiosyncrasies. We saw in Chapter 3, 'The hallmarks of excellence', how many of Vocational Training's cardinal sins and virtues lie in the domains of beliefs, values, mission and motivation. Glance back now, and notice also how extensively the language used by the Course Organisers to describe them is permeated with value-laden phrases of their own. Here are some examples taken from replies to my survey:

"Ignorance is a challenge, not a threat";
"Not prepared to widen horizons";
"Brutalized by hospital medicine";
"Unable or unwilling to reveal own vulnerability";
"Do not exploit others to gratify own emotional needs";
"Fire in the belly!";

"Have to be spoon-fed";
"Unwilling to involve themselves with their hearts";
"Has the will to strive towards optimum standards".

If we were to ask these Course Organisers how they first became aware of these so-called "attitude problems", they might reply, "I don't know, it was the way he spoke about . . .; it just made me uneasy". They would have been sensing incongruence between their *own* values and those inferred from the Trainees' value-laden language.

So: "Listen out for value-laden phrases as minimal cues to possible learning needs." But beware; there is a danger here, summarised in Juvenal's well-known paradox, *Quis custodiet ipsos custodes?* – Who is to guard the guards themselves? Noticing unusually prominent value cues in another person's remarks brings one's own values in that area rushing self-defensively to the surface. Who is to appraise the values of the value-appraisers? When value incongruence is detected it is wrong to assume that the origin of the misalignment is necessarily the other party. Value-laden phrases are a trickier learning cue to deal with than the speech censoring already described because of the cognitive dissonance they induce in the listener. It behoves the teacher to register his own cognitive dissonance – evoked feelings, for instance, of antagonism, bewilderment or strong sympathy – and allow it to prompt a re-examination of his own learning needs.

An undue proportion of value-laden words and phrases indicates that the speaker's cognitive dissonance has been aroused, but is probably being dealt with in a maladaptive non-learning way. It implies either that the self-image is locally vulnerable, or else that the educational environment offers too little in the way of 'safe insecurity' for learning to occur.

Imagery and metaphor

Periodically, the prosaic exchanges that typify most of our tutorial dialogues are punctuated with an unexpected flight, if not into poetry, at least into imagery and metaphor. For instance: the patient whose depression is being discussed may unexpectedly be described as resembling "a record stuck in the groove, and a scratched record at that." Or a Trainee unhappy about relationships with senior colleagues might venture, "It makes you wonder what it took to kill off the dinosaurs!" A sudden shift like this in the power of the language has implications similar to, but possibly more intense than, the value-laden phrases described above. It indicates a value system feeling itself beleaguered. We learn that the first speaker is irritated by the patient and longs to administer a firm therapeutic nudge. The second's murderous intent and appeal to cosmic vengeance may be dismissed as fantasy, but the underlying resentment is nonetheless real and strong. When people resort to symbolic imagery, it is often because they need to assert the rectitude of their own views particularly urgently. Metaphorical language has on the listener the disarming effect of suspending disbelief, of numbing any inclination to be objectively critical, much as a good story does on its reader. A speaker giving way to imagery (here goes!) is like a bird that, by elaborate and dramatic flutterings, hopes to distract a predator's attention from her nest and its helpless fledglings.

Turn back for a moment to the preceding section on 'Value-laden phrases', the second and third paragraphs (p. 142). They are written in over-blown language, even for me! And yet . . . at the time I wrote them I felt the ideas they express (1) mattered, and (2) might encounter resistance on the part of the reader, who might therefore think badly of me. Aware of my own strong self-justifying tendency, I sidestep criticism (from which I might learn) by using imagery to switch the level of debate to a more emotive and less objective plane.

Teachers need to remain alert to the sub-text of symbolism and the striking image; it may be the start of a trail leading to the well-spring of a pupil's motivation.

PARA-LINGUISTIC CUES

So that we maintain a sense of direction, let me briefly recapitulate where this discussion of minimal cues is leading. Whatever the educational agenda dictated by curriculum- and assessment-based teaching, people's day-to-day and moment-to-moment learning is governed by an Inner Apprentice, working to an 'Inner Curriculum' of its own highly personal learning needs. The Inner Apprentice signals what it currently wants to learn by allowing a variety of minimal cues to leak out. The learner may be fully aware of *some* of his or her learning needs, but not all; many are not signalled consciously. A necessary supplement to a teacher's skills, therefore, is the ability to recognise and bring into consciousness the subtler indications of the Inner Curriculum, so that it can be identified and in due course addressed.

So far we have considered only language-based cues. I have tried to indicate how the words learners use contain more information than teachers may credit. The words mean more than they say. In order to retrieve the Inner Apprentice's signals, the stream of speech has to be attended to in a different way. We have to listen out for different things – the 'off-the-cuff' remarks, the things that are *not* said and *nearly* said, the detailed choice of vocabulary. It's as if there is an extra channel of communication embedded beneath the surface meaning. We have to turn ourselves into a kind of 'Teletext decoder', able to reveal the extra information transmitted in the gaps between successive pictures on the TV screen.

If we now turn to the remaining minimal cues, those not based on the sense of the spoken word, our consideration can be more concise. They are special cases of the non-verbal communication we are already familiar with. 'Para-linguistic cues' are also based on language, but on its overall sound rather than on the exact meaning. You could spot para-linguistic cues even if the speaker spoke a foreign language you did not understand.

Delivery

'Delivery' here means what an actor means by it – the way the voice sounds and the way it is projected. Like actors, we have in our kit a range of tones of voice, and we use particular voices in particular situations and for particular purposes. We each have a voice for being 'business-like' in; another for being 'relaxed' in; others for being 'cautious', or 'enthusiastic', or 'light-hearted', 'defensive', 'confident', 'bored', 'urgent'. The discriminating qualities include:

> Pitch – high or low; soprano, alto, tenor or bass; falsetto or chalumeau; monotone or with rise and fall;
>
> Pace – fast or slow; constant or varying in speed; getting faster or slowing down; rhythmical or sporadic;
>
> Volume – soft or loud; crescendo or diminuendo; constant volume, or with moments of greater or lesser emphasis.

A change in delivery, even if the subject matter seems not to alter, and especially if there seems to be incongruence between subject and tone of voice, may indicate a significant change in the speaker's inner world for the teacher to be aware of.

Turbulence

The energy of a passage of speech can be rated on a 'turbulence' scale ranging from measured tranquillity to extreme agitation. A river passing over rapids becomes broken up into 'white water', implying the presence of boulders on its bed. In the same way the stream of speech tends to become turbulent when some invisible obstacle disturbs the speaker. Delivery becomes erratic, fractured, restless, with abrupt changes of pace, pitch and volume. The voice may sound tense. There may also be signs of physical restlessness, with frequent shifts of position and rapid eye movements. At such moments the listener's antennae should be set to maximum sensitivity, and close attention paid to clues to a possible cause.

Micro-emotions

Sometimes one can detect short-lived but definitely genuine flickers of real emotion in a speaker's remarks, remarks that someone else might have uttered with equanimity. Certain topics have the power to stir up old memories or re-stimulate old feelings. So the attuned ear may hear a distinct huskiness or catch in the voice as a doctor says, "She looked after her dying mother *really* well", accompanied perhaps by down-cast gaze and a moistening eye. The voice of a doctor who "simply could *not* get the hospital to take the patient!" may betray a note of real anger, confirmed by a clenched fist. Or the gritted teeth through which another complains that he has had to see "too many extra patients today" may indicate that on this occasion he feels more than a token resentment.

Micro-emotions of this sort may suggest an inappropriate intrusion of unresolved psychological business, resolution of which might be a legitimate educational goal.

NON-VERBAL CUES

Internal search

People exhibit a particular cluster of non-verbal signs when they are momentarily occupied in some serious thinking. (In fact, if you pause in your reading at this point and try to imagine how people look when they're doing some serious thinking, you will yourself exhibit this behaviour!)

This is 'internal search'. Its signs are:

(1) Sudden bodily stillness, perhaps only for an instant, but sometimes producing a state of catatonia lasting several seconds. The thinker freezes even in mid-gesture; and

(2) Changes in gaze. The eyes either
(a) move around very rapidly, as when dreaming, while the thinker scans numerous memories;
(b) remain steadily fixed in one direction, either upwards and

147

usually to the left (if the thinker is accessing visual memories), or downwards and to the right (if a feeling is being recalled); or

(c) become still and de-focussed, the thinker looking, as it were, either inwards or into the far distance, oblivious to the surroundings.

If you have any video recordings of yourself consulting, internal search is easily and frequently spotted in patients, particularly during the history-taking phase of the consultation. Its significance there is the same as its significance in an educational setting – the thinker is interrogating memory to see if it contains the information circumstances presently require.

Internal search indicates that the mental task being carried out is a complex one, needing significant time for completion; or that what is being considered matters; or that the thinker knows himself to be on thin ice and needing to choose his next words with care. At all events the inner-directed teacher should attend closely to what is said immediately after a period of internal search. Either the requisite information will have been found or it will not. If not, a learning need exists and cognitive dissonance will ensue. Internal search followed by signs of cognitive dissonance indicates a significant learning opportunity.

Energy shifts

When listening to people speak, we often notice what might be called their 'energy level' – a greater or lesser quality of urgency, of animation, interest, involvement, passion. At the same time we may pick up signs that the energy is emotionally-charged – hints that the speaker feels moved, angry, excited, embarrassed, amused, tense, and so on. These variations in energy and affect indicate what playwrights call 'sub-text', the deeper and possibly truer meaning beneath the surface sense of the words. They allow us to estimate why and to what extent the speaker is committed to what he is saying, how much it matters to him, how he feels about it.

Energy level can fluctuate rapidly in quality and intensity during the course of even a brief conversation. Signs that an energy shift is occurring include adjustments of physical posture, changes in eye contact and hand gesturing, and indications of tension in the vocal delivery. We are all perfectly familiar with non-verbal communications of this sort; what may nonetheless bear emphasising is their significance as minimal cues to the hovering presence of a learner's Inner Curriculum. Most of the time the energy level and emotional charge of speech are appropriate to its content. Sometimes, however, they don't quite seem to add up. We may feel surprised when powerful events are described apathetically, or mundane ones with passion. The reason for some particular emotional colouring may not be at first apparent. Such brief moments of incongruence between content on one hand, and energy and affect on the other suggest some degree of cognitive dissonance on the part of the speaker. Fine-tuning of the listening ear and sharpening of the watching eye may identify an underlying learning need.

Displacement activities

Experts on animal behaviour tell us than when an animal is evenly torn between two conflicting needs or instincts it either 'freezes' or performs a displacement activity irrelevant to both. A cat, uncertain whether to approach a stranger to be stroked or retreat in case of danger, may instead start to wash. In people, too, displacement activities indicate the presence of cognitive dissonance. Trivial examples include fiddling with a pen, scratching one's nose, making an unneeded cup of coffee. In the tutorial context, conflict between the desire to learn and the wish to remain unchallenged might result in highjacking discussion with an abrupt change of subject, 'remembering' some urgent unfinished business, 'forgetting' to turn on the video recorder, or (sacrilegious thought!) having another bash at assessment. Displacement activities like this are the behavioural equivalents of the linguistic non sequiturs described earlier.

Occasionally displacement activities can assume distractingly impressive proportions, e.g. going on extended but irrelevant courses, or undertaking complex audits and projects to answer questions hardly worth the asking.

Gaze

Mutual gaze between speakers obeys a highly complex and largely unconscious choreography. Eye contact is used to punctuate speech, to regulate the handover from one speaker to another, to convey culture-dependent messages about status, and so on. But although it may be hard to define 'normal' gaze between two people, both can easily tell when the unspoken rules are broken. The eye signs of internal search may break gaze for long enough to be noticeable, but they are recognizably different from the 'avoidance of eye contact' suggesting shiftiness or the 'downcast' gaze of the depressed or preoccupied. Excessively prolonged direct gaze – 'staring out' – has a challenging quality of "come and get me if you can".

Incongruities of gaze often appear when one of the conversing parties is experiencing cognitive dissonance. Gaze disruption is a behavioural equivalent of the speech-censoring omissions and hesitations described in the earlier account of linguistic cues.

TRAINING ONESELF TO RECOGNISE MINIMAL CUES

> I am a camera with its shutter open, quite passive, recording, not thinking. Recording the man shaving at the window opposite and the woman in the kimono washing her hair. Some day, all this will have to be developed, carefully printed, fixed.

> Christopher Isherwood, *Goodbye to Berlin*

I have given lengthy consideration to the minimal cues of cognitive dissonance in order to try and bring about a shift in perception – the teacher's perception of what observations matter during the course of a particular learning session. I am suggesting that a different kind of data is worth paying one's best attention to. The difference lies not in the novelty of the minimal cues, for they are all part of familiar everyday conversation. What here is different is their meaning and the educational use to which they can be put. My suggestion is that a teacher sensitive to these signals from a pupil's Inner Apprentice, and willing to follow the path they chart through the Inner Curriculum, will find it easier to focus attention on areas of here-and-now relevance.

Training oneself to make use of minimal educational cues is a matter of consciousness-raising, a matter of 'getting one's eye and ear in', of sensitising oneself to notice what had previously passed unnoticed. The exercises I propose are 'practice in noticing'. A word of caution: picking up on the minimal cues in a tutorial is not an end in itself, but rather (in Isherwood's "*I am a camera*" metaphor) the imprinting of a latent image subsequently to be developed, printed and fixed at the right time. To change the analogy, minimal cues indicate the tutorial's sub-text, but that sub-text need not always be read aloud; silently will do. The teacher's own Inner Apprentice can be trusted to draw attention to the cues that matter. What matters will get noticed. What's noticed doesn't *have* to be addressed; but what's *not* noticed can never be.

I remember as a schoolboy playing 'noughts and crosses' ('Tic Tac Toe'), and being shown for the first time how you need never lose, and can always win against an opponent who doesn't know the key blocking move. Delighted, I would pester people to play me. Luckily, the novelty soon wore off. The thing is, with minimal cue tracking as with noughts and crosses, once you know the trick you can never again naively play the game.

Training exercise 1

Here is a series of awareness-raising questions designed to heighten your powers of observation. Try to answer them as accurately as possible. Some call only for introspection; others require you to experiment a little. The phrasing of the questions assumes that you are a Trainer familiar with an individual Trainee. If this is not the case, reframe them as necessary.

(1) How do I usually manage to tell what my Trainee's current area of concern is?

(2) What are the tell-tale signs indicating that the Trainee's stated problem is not the underlying one that *really* concerns him?

(3) How often do I find myself wondering exactly what the Trainee means?

(4) What kind of information do I usually have to press him for?

(5) How often, when my Trainee is describing something he has done, do I find myself wishing he would hurry up and get to the point?

(6) What occasions can I recall when I have bridled at some of the attitudes and values I think I have detected in what my Trainee has said?

(7) How can I tell when my Trainee is unsure of his own knowledge base?

(8) Can I recall any particularly vivid images or metaphors the Trainee has used recently?

(9) What adjectives describe the Trainee's usual tone of voice?

(10) If I surreptitiously watch people around me, how easy is it to spot signs of 'internal search'?

(11) What are my own favourite displacement activities during the course of a working day?

(12) What are the Trainee's favourite displacement activities?

(13) What proportion of people's speech seems to carry hints about their emotional state?

(14) In what circumstances do I consciously control the direction and intensity of my own gaze?

Training exercise 2

Make a video recording of any or all of the following: yourself consulting with patients; someone else (Trainee or colleague) consulting with patients; a tutorial session in which you are involved as either teacher or learner. Figure 7.2 consists of a check-list of the various cues to cognitive dissonance. If necessary, re-read the preceding sections until you are happy that you can recognise them. Then watch your chosen video. Whenever you think you see an example of a particular cue, put a tick in the corresponding box. It doesn't matter whether you are 'right' or not: after all, who other than you is going to tell? The exercise's value lies in the effect it has on your own ability to perceive oases of import amidst the sands of inconsequence.

Perception on the verge of action

The central thesis of this book is that *people are intrinsically self-educating, as long as the right information is presented in the right way at the right time.* For a teacher, the ability to track minimal cues as they unfold within a tutorial setting is a great help in judging the 'right time' for making an educational intervention. Minimal cues also give pretty good pointers as to what is likely to prove 'right' (i.e. truly mutative) information. Paying high-quality attention to minimal cues helps bring both teacher and learner to a state of 'perception on the verge of action'. How to make effective use of this heightened perception is the topic of the next chapter.

CURTAIN RAISERS	
GAMBITS	
SPEECH CENSORING (1) Omissions Distortions Generalizations	
SPEECH CENSORING (2) Hesitations Procrastinations	
SPEECH CENSORING (3) Non sequiturs	
VALUE–LADEN PHRASES	
TURBULENCE	
MICRO–EMOTIONS	
INTERNAL SEARCH	
ENERGY SHIFTS	
GAZE DISTURBANCES	

Figure 7.2 'Cognitive dissonance cues' training check list

Chapter 8

The point of kairos

However certain our expectation
The moment foreseen may be unexpected
When it arrives.

T. S. Eliot, *Murder in the Cathedral*

Learn to recognize beginnings.

John Heider, *The Tao of Leadership*

'Thought For The Day', the nub, the crucial moment, the moment of truth, – call it what you will. Once or twice (seldom more) in any worthwhile tutorial encounter a critical moment comes when Something Significant is poised to happen. Various portents and forces have been coaxed into conjunction. The topic is relevant. The patient has in some way challenged the doctor's competence. The case contains potential depths which the learner is nearly (but not quite) equipped to explore. Discussion has led gently but firmly to a point where the depths can be glimpsed. The learner, hesitant and perhaps caught a little off-balance, is nonetheless confident enough that support is available, and wants to proceed. The teacher is reading the learner's state of mind sufficiently accurately to judge when to push, when to stand back, and when to assist. Such a moment, when the course of subsequent learning is there for the changing, is the point of *kairos*.

Kairos is the Greek word for the right time for action, the propitious moment when events cry out to be taken in hand. It is interesting that the Greeks had a word for it, while we, for all our educational sophistication, have not. And yet every Trainer I have spoken to recognises not only the phenomenon but also its crucial importance for the effectiveness of one-to-one teaching. As the tale of Rumpelstiltskin reminds us, to know something's name is to begin to control it. So may I be forgiven for proposing 'kairos' as the name of these educational cross-roads, and 'kairotic' as the adjective to describe them?

Alan Bennett, in one of his wry plays about our ridiculous frailties, has a Yorkshirewoman say, with mouthwashed vowels, "My stomach's on a knife-edge – it could go either way!" At the point of kairos, so could cognitive dissonance go either way. Handled maladaptively, it will dissipate in contortions of self-justification or turn in upon itself in unmerited self-abnegation, as the E. M. Forster passages quoted in Chapter 6 describe. The potentially transforming voltage will leak away and will have to be regenerated another day. But handled with gentle persistence the discomfort of cognitive dissonance can be converted into transformational energy. The teacher's skill is to secure this metamorphosis less by luck than by design.

Cox and Theilgard's book *Mutative Metaphors in Psychotherapy* [1] uses the same word 'kairos' to describe moments of similar potential energy in the context of psychoanalysis. Their theme is how a listening therapist can resonate to the poetic overtones in a patient's story until its reverberations call forth new and insightful harmonics of therapeutic response. A therapist, they remind us (op. cit. p. 105),

> must not thrust his own preformed imagery upon a patient who is cautiously seeking to express the inexpressible. But neither must he withhold (insight) if a patient is searching for that which needs to be called into being . . . This is a threshold phenomenon of the greatest finesse. . . Discerning the optimal time for an intervention is something which may improve with experience. But the therapist is always likely to feel that his interventions could have been better located and more felicitously timed. Energy spent in discerning the moment of *kairos* is never wasted. It is *the* moment in which to speak or to be silent. Furthermore, if it is genuinely kairotic, the patient will also be aware that it is *the* moment, and he will look no further for the thing itself.

The same authors adduce others in support of this increasingly important theme. Hammer [2], reviewing the depth and timing of interpretations, suggests that,

> In terms of depth there is more or less agreement that the surface of the unconscious is the level to be sought. One communicates to the patient what the patient is *almost* ready to see for himself, that which is just outside awareness. . . Thus, by drawing the near, but unseen, closer to its ultimate elucidation, we put within the patient's grasp that which is just beyond it.

Likewise Freud [3] talks about the 'navel' of a dream,

the spot where it reaches down into the unknown.

(Lest the parallels between education and therapy give offence, let me make clear that I am not suggesting that to be a Trainee is to be psychiatrically disturbed! Rather the converse is true: psychotherapy is more a special case of education than of therapeutics. The point of both is that through interaction with an empathetic outsider impediments to personal fulfilment can be overcome.)

So at a tutorial's point of kairos the Trainee has come to perceive with maximum clarity the essence of some shortcoming or difficulty, and feels most hungry for help with it. There is maximal curiosity, maximal sense of personal involvement and maximal resolve to learn. Both learner and teacher are aware that this is the pivotal point to which the previous discussion has inexorably been leading; the minds of both are sharply focused on the same key issue. The Trainee's Inner Apprentice has identified the nub, and the teacher's willingness to be guided by his pupil's minimal cues has led him simultaneously to the same realisation. Both may have a sense of 'tunnel vision' as inessential detail falls away. The Trainee feels a strange mixture of vulnerability, because some previously concealed inadequacy has been revealed, and excitement, because the educational environment is trustworthy and assistance is at hand. The teacher in turn feels most strongly a sense of solidarity and empathy with his pupil. He knows that now – not a moment ago, not in a moment yet, but *now* – a skilled intervention will have its most valuable effect. He also feels an elation tinged with anxiety, lest the opportunity be missed. The Trainee's Inner Apprentice is revealed like a nocturnal animal caught in a car's headlights; depending on the teacher's approach it may dash for the safety of concealment or be coaxed into new confidence.

Dead Poets Society, the 1989 movie starring Robin Williams as John Keating, a charismatic English teacher in an oppressively curriculum-dominated school in Vermont, is a film about kairos. Keating's motto is *'Carpe diem'* – 'Seize the day!' "Make your lives extraordinary", he enjoins his astonished class. Subversively (the regime obliges him to be subversive) he alerts his pupils to their own potential destinies. Because they sense that Keating is no flash manipulator but genuinely desires their betterment, each pupil is inspired to follow through on the opportunity and risks 'seizing the day'. One, disobeying his father, discovers a talent for acting; another finds the courage to pursue a love affair, another to challenge the authority of a martinet headmaster. Because this is Hollywood, the successes are triumphant and the failures fatally catastrophic. We must not be intimidated by the risk of such extremities. Even in the mundane setting of a General Practice tutorial it is possible – essential – to know the day, and to seize the kairotic moment.

The purpose of a tutorial is not to teach. The purpose of a tutorial is to reach a point of kairos. A point of kairos, if successfully reached, will inevitably be followed by effective teaching and sound learning, because the perceptual and awareness-raising processes that will have generated it are the same processes that will not allow it to be wasted.

This chapter is an exploration of the kairotic moment in a one-to-one tutorial: how to recognise it and how to set up conditions favourable to its emergence.

TUTORIAL RHYTHMS – 'FLOW' AND 'FLUTTER'

If asked afterwards to describe what occurred during a tutorial encounter, both parties usually reply in terms of what topic was discussed, what problem was identified, what was learned. Descriptions of the tutorial's process, (as opposed to its content), if verbalised at all, tend to be in analytical 'curricular' language of objectives, models and strategies. Yet if the participants tune in to the tutorial experience at the time it is occurring, the more powerful sensation is not of studied analysis but of 'things being in motion'. Thoughts come and go; energy levels shift; questions suggest themselves unbidden, and answers come impromptu; significant ideas and moments of emotional charge alternate with each other and with periods of free-wheeling. Teacher and learner each seem to be dancing from one focus of attention to another, seldom in step with each other. Understanding and order may ultimately result, but they may not always seem to emerge in a logical and ordered way.

Yet the tutorial's pulsing movement – its choreography – is fundamental to its outcome, and is neither random nor mysterious. The focus of attention dances to two simultaneous rhythms, one with a slow beat and one faster. The slow rhythm we can think of as a cyclical 'tidal flow', in which educational impetus gradually builds to a maximum and then recedes. Superimposed on this is a more rapid 'butterfly flutter'; smaller excursions and distractions occur, carrying the attention briefly away from and back to the session's emergent themes. As the point of kairos is approached, the 'thought rhythms' of learner and teacher become more and more synchronised and attuned to each other. (The reader with a nose for metaphor might see parallels between this and other mutually satisfying intimate human encounters!)

The tutorial's tidal cycle: 'might–should–must–does–did'

Regardless of starting point or topic, the tutorial's energy can be felt to undergo a slow tidal movement, a building up followed by a falling away. At first the learner's educational needs for that day may be hard to discern, but as discussion proceeds the real agenda becomes more and more clear, more and more insistent. Like an ocean responding to the powerful influences of currents, celestial bodies and local geography, the force for learning gathers itself progressively into a ground-swell, then into a tidal surge, then individual waves, until at the kairotic moment of the tutorial's high water mark a particular wave of insight breaks on the day's particular shore. Then the tidal energy subsides; surf that was powerful and exhilarating recedes and rejoins the amorphous sea, to regather and come ashore again on the next tide.

The focus of tutorial attention undergoes just such a tidal cycle. At the start of a session of potential learning there may be mixed feelings of curiosity, expectancy and some anxiety, the more so if the topic has not been rigorously pre-ordained. Soon, however, there may come into the teacher's mind an inkling of some lesson that might be learned, some educational need that might be inferred from the material so far presented. The temptation to formulate an early educational focus is strong but risky. Both teacher and pupil may experience a welcome relief from anxiety if both agree at an early stage that "This is what we'll concentrate on today, then." Unfortunately the Inner Curriculum seldom asserts itself so rapidly or so conveniently, and any short-lived relief is soon replaced by increasing frustration. Frustration is even more likely if either party mounts a favourite hobby-horse, for even a jointly owned hobby-horse soon tires. It is usually preferable for the teacher to defer an early formulation and give full attention instead to detecting the indicative minimal cues, discussed earlier, until their message is unequivocal.

When the minimal cues begin to indicate some potential educational focus – some learning that '*might*' occur – deft assistance, using particularly awareness-raising questions, can lead discussion with mounting inexorability through a stage of what '*should*' to what '*must*' occur. The point when learning that '*must*' occur becomes what '*does*' occur is the point of kairos. If the focus has been well-judged and its implications skilfully followed-through, the learning that does occur is then consolidated as an enduring knowledge gain that '*did*' occur. *Might–should–must–does–did*: this repeating tidal cycle is, I believe, a more authentic model of education's fundamental process than the traditional paradigm of objectives–methods–assessment. A single tutorial session, limited by concentration span, usually seems to accommodate one or at the most two tidal cycles.

From the learner's point of view the tutorial's tidal rhythm might begin in the safe shallows of discursive discussion. As the depths are sensed, increasing cognitive dissonance accompanies the progression from *might* towards *should* and *must*. If the inevitable insecurity contrives to be safe enough, at the point of kairos insight and motivation arise in sufficient degree to acknowledge, confront and resolve the identified knowledge gap. Cognitive resonance indicates when learning successfully *does* occur.

Butterfly flutter

The path is seldom smooth from the tutorial's initial low-key generalities to its charge-carrying point of kairos. Superimposed on the tidal cycle are smaller precessions of interest. Along the way the attention of learner, pupil, or both, flits erratically from point to interesting point like a butterfly amongst flowers. It settles fleetingly on a promising bloom, only to flutter away apparently oblivious to the nectar that lay at hand had it but stayed and probed a little longer. Moments of insight and real learning are haphazardly interspersed with distractions and diversions. The difficulty is to tell one from the other at the time. Both parties find themselves wondering, "Does this matter? Is it relevant? What ought we to be concentrating on here?" Then a moment later confidence returns: "Ah, now we're on the right lines. There's a really important point here; let's deal with it thoroughly."

REACHING THE POINT OF KAIROS

We can now draw together a number of themes already developed, and use them to chart a course through sometimes difficult educational terrain. Let's consider the tutorial process from the point of view of the principal protagonist – the learner's Inner Apprentice. The tutorial exists mainly – solely – to provide the Inner Apprentice with scope for expression and learning.

No matter how the tutorial's starting topic is decided – pre-selected or opportunistically – the Inner Apprentice will quickly identify its own priority learning needs according to an Inner Curriculum, and will begin to test the educational environment's capacity to satisfy them. This it does by drawing the learner's attention, unconsciously and involuntarily at first, to some particular aspects of the topic rather than to others. The learner finds, without knowing quite why, that certain features claim his attention in preference to others; certain questions occur to him while others do not; certain ideas puzzle and intrigue more than others; certain thoughts seem worth expressing while others pass unheeded. This process of 'automatic selection' is not random; it indicates that the Inner Apprentice has begun to identify what Inner Curricular learning needs are on today's agenda.

An example: Trainer and Trainee are discussing paediatric surveillance, using the Trainee's recent consultation with a mother and child as a focus. The Trainee breaks off from discussing how to test for squint to ask the Trainer, "Do you know this mother? I couldn't seem to get through to her." The Inner Apprentice has realised that of greater immediate relevance than the squint is the issue of maternal behaviour and the doctor–patient relationship. In order to achieve this re-prioritising, it has 'made' this apparent non sequitur of a question form in the Trainee's mind. The question deserves neither to be ignored nor cursorily answered, but rather explored by such a response as "What prompts you to ask?"

For the teacher, the tutorial's agenda is to 'read the Inner Apprentice's mind' – to discover gently but systematically what leads the learner's attention to move (either by tidal flow or butterfly flutter) in the directions that it does.

The teacher's role

Two complementary skills are of value to the teacher in fashioning an educational crunch point. The first is the ability to choreograph the tutorial's tidal flow, that rise of curiosity from initial generalities to an intense and significant crux. The second is to be able to keep sensitive and balanced control of the inevitable flutter, so that pursuit of the tutorial's important themes is not for too long interrupted by incidental distractions, however beguiling.

The first skill, tidal management, can be improved by the Socratic 'answer begets question' method of dialectic described in Chapter 1, combined with monitoring the minimal cues catalogued in Chapter 7. 'Flutter control', the second skill, is primarily achieved by the judicious use of the awareness-raising question.

Neo-Socratic style

At this point, it may help to refresh your memory of the section on Socrates in Chapter 1, pages 22 to 24.

In his dialogues Socrates showed himself to be a master of tidal management, from whom we now do well to learn. Figures 1.2 and 1.3 (pages 25 and 26) summarise his uniquely effective method. The educational dialectic begins by agreeing what topic is to be its starting point. It then attempts through questioning to discover precisely what is in the minds of the interlocutors as they struggle to express their understanding in mere words. This process of *elenchus* being sustained, it is inevitable that the limits of knowledge of one or other (not necessarily the identified learner!) will eventually be reached. The teacher's role is, by clarifying and questioning, to establish whatever deficits in knowledge base, assumptions and values are currently limiting the learner's effectiveness or understanding.

For Socrates, the turning-point in a dialogue came when his probing questions reduced the other to confess a state of helpless ignorance – *aporia*. Despite his protestations to the contrary, this often seemed the moment for Socrates to score easy points, showing off his own virtuoso intellect to the delight both of himself and of the onlookers. Thus embarrassed, the student's all too frequent response must have been not insight but resentment; true learning sacrificed upon the altar of vainglory. Socratic aporia is not quite the point of kairos we seek. Kairos is free of any compulsive need by the teacher to impose his own diagnosis or remedy unless genuinely asked to; it is truly learner-centred. At the point of kairos ignorance is reframed as a 'passion to know'. And it needs to be the learner's *own* passion. A skilled teacher may be able to foster passion in a student; a well-prepared teacher can if required then supply information for which the student has become passionate; and an impassioned teacher can model what it is to take delight in learning. But the point of kairos is no place for second-hand passion: had Socrates understood this he might have been spared the hemlock.

In Chapter 1 I listed the ground-rules of Socratic dialogue. It is worth revisiting them here as, shorn of Socrates' egotism, they still offer useful principles for contemporary seekers after educational impact.

Agreed agenda and definitions

Logically, the need for two debating persons to agree on what they are discussing and why they are bothering seems unarguable. It does however appear that Socrates – whether intentionally or not we shall never know – usually either imposed his own agenda or else coerced that of his interlocutor, by his own strength of personality, into a form Socrates knew he could dominate. Socrates' inclination to use teaching as a vehicle for self-aggrandisement was not an endearing characteristic, and it remains one for us to guard against. Translating into contemporary jargon, we should say that the teacher's secret agenda should have low priority, while the learner's secret agenda – his Inner Curriculum – is to be paramount. Part of the teacher's professionalism should reside in his ability consciously to identify, and consciously to subordinate, teaching objectives dearer to his own heart than his pupil's.

Questions, not statements

Socrates was probably the first teacher systematically to eschew didacticism. He knew that, wherever truth may reside, the individual postulant best approaches it from his own precepts and by his own route. So, asking is more effective than telling. Socrates' personal style was to 'let each answer beg the next question': whatever view the learner proposed was to have its validity tested by challenging its implications. As an educational technique, Socratic questioning is an improvement on dogmatic insistence that "teacher knows best". Yet there is a form of pseudo-Socratic question that essentially keeps asking, with a thinly-veiled sneer, "I see; so you seriously maintain, do you, . . . ?", and which palpably digs a pit for the increasingly beleaguered student to fall into. Defensiveness and resentment are the inevitable consequences. The Socratic question is an excellent educational device as long as it is genuinely conducive to exploration of the learner's inner assumptive world. But it is not the only, nor indeed the best, such device. The awareness-raising question, which we shall shortly consider in more detail, may be more respectful and therefore more effective.

Minimal cues

If we allow the premise that, left to its own devices, the Inner Apprentice will direct the learner's attention to those aspects of the issue from which he can best learn, it becomes apparent how important it is for the teacher to keep constant track of minimal cues during a tutorial. For minimal behavioural cues constitute the outwardly observable indications of where, on a moment by moment basis, the learner's attention is located. Minimal cues reveal the 'state of the tutorial tide'.

In Chapter 7 we reviewed the various ways – verbal, para-verbal and non-verbal – in which minimal cues betray the cognitive dissonance of a learner who finds his own knowledge base to be inadequate and who therefore needs to learn. Pointers to the Inner Curriculum reside in:

- the learner's opening gambit and curtain-raisers, particular if their messages seem to be conflicting;
- speech censoring, i.e. omissions, distortions, generalisations, procrastinations and non sequiturs;
- value-laden phrases;
- verbal and non-verbal turbulence;
- micro-emotions and energy shifts;
- internal search and other disturbances of gaze indicating moments of more than average importance to the thinker.

Safe insecurity

'Tidal management' in the tutorial uses a neo-Socratic, i.e. benevolently challenging, questioning style to reveal the learner's curiosity and intensify it until the nub of the issue is clearly recognised and expressed. Neo-Socratic questioning, designed deliberately to unsettle but not devastate the learner, is often appropriate in the early stages of a tutorial. Cognitive dissonance must be generated and intensified, while at the same time being kept within tolerable limits. Learning occurs best under conditions of 'safe insecurity'. Unless the learner appreciates that his existing knowledge store is inadequate there is no incentive to modify it. Yet the teacher's questions must be non-hostile, his challenges clearly well-intentioned. If the confrontation is too great or too aggressive there is a risk of maladaptive retreat into entrenchment and self-justification. Neo-Socratic questioning, while respecting the learner's vulnerability, challenges whatever knowledge, assumptions and values currently seem to be limiting effectiveness – but it challenges them gently. The way to ensure gentleness is for the teacher to remain unobtrusively attuned to the learner's minimal cues, using them to judge the timing and phrasing of his questions and interventions.

To keep track of minimal cues requires the teacher to remain less than usually preoccupied with his own internal thoughts, and more receptive to indications of the learner's Inner Curriculum. It helps for a teacher constantly to be asking himself:

> *What is the learner's attention on*
> *at this precise moment? And how can I tell?*

AWARENESS-CENTRED TEACHING

In Vocational Training a distinction is often made between Trainer-centred and Trainee-centred styles of teaching. Trainer-centred teaching relies mainly on traditional educational processes of telling, instructing, suggesting and recommending. Its deep structure is 'education as revelation', elaborated in this book's opening chapter and encapsulated in the slogan 'teacher knows best'. The Trainee-centred approach, on the other hand, evangelically preached by a growing band of subversives, is a form of 'education as quest'. Here the slogan is 'let them work it out for themselves'. This philosophy underpins a teaching style which encourages experimentation, guessing, trial and error, learning from one's mistakes. Both styles do of course have their merits. In their pure forms, neither is self-sufficient.

Besides being Trainer- or Trainee-centred a teaching style can be positioned along a second and unrelated axis – 'concept-centred' versus 'awareness-centred'. By 'concept-centred' I mean a style in which the teacher structures his contribution to be substantially in accordance with cherished concepts such as 'core curriculum', 'aims and objectives', 'self-directed learning', rating scales, models and paradigms. A concept-centred teacher 'teaches like the theory tells him'. The awareness-centred teacher, on the other hand, prefers to follow his nose. His is a more experiential style: he draws what guidance he needs from the cues he detects in the immediate encounter. He finds 'teaching to the concept' not so much wrong as unrewarding. Concept-centred teaching tries, but frequently fails, to coerce the learner's experience into a structure and sequence it may not comfortably fit. Not surprisingly, there is no such thing as a bespoke straight-jacket. Through awareness-centred teaching the Trainee learns through noticing, realising and acknowledging. The teacher is judged by how skilfully he can help his Trainee to notice, realise and acknowledge whatever insights he is presently minded to acquire.

As far as I can see, the Inner Apprentice prefers awareness-centred teaching. Concepts and abstractions either go over its head or get up its nose. (And even as I write I am aware of how ineffective this the written word is at communicating with you the reader's own Inner Apprentice: those potentially most sympathetic to what I am saying may find themselves most alienated by the way print constrains me to say it – a poignant paradox.)

We first met the Inner Apprentice during an awareness-centred golf lesson in Chapter 5. The coach there confined himself to exploring the pupil's immediate physical sensations by asking awareness-raising questions (ARQs) – what?, when?, where?, how much? Non-judgemental questioning led the pupil to become engrossed in just those aspects of performance where close attention would lead to improvement. The coach resisted the temptation to weigh in with theories, advice or instruction. These were saved until a suitable lull in inner-directed curiosity when the pupil's attention became spontaneously disengaged from the task of swinging the golf club. The coach's expertise resided in his ability to ask ARQs in such a way that the learner's own unconscious mind selected the learning agenda and directed the focus of attention. We concluded then that 'People are intrinsically self-educating, as long as the right information is provided in the right way at the right time'. The 'right information' means that for which the learner's here-and-now attention finds itself spontaneously hungry. The 'right way' means non-judgementally, safely yet uncompromisingly, and engaging the learner's sustained interest. And the 'right time' is the point of kairos.

The route to kairos is paved with ARQs.

ARQs in the tutorial

The raw materials of golf are club selection, the swing, the impact, the flight of the ball, whether straight and true, scuffed, pulled or sliced, hazard avoidance, recovery from adverse positions, deftness of short game, cultivation of match temperament . . . Maybe the reason so many GPs play golf is that the game involves similar skills to those they already employ, invisibly and metaphorically, in their consulting rooms! 'Inner Golf' coaching and coaching the Inner Apprentice are alike in that the process involves raising non-judgemental here-and-now awareness. However when coaching for General Practice the focus is not so much on the learner's bodily sensations and physical orientation as on his stream of consciousness as it meanders amongst an inner cognitive and affective landscape. Specifically, we are interested in the learner's thoughts, ideas, images, associations, reactions, micro-emotions – the running commentary that forms inside his mind as a piece of work is reviewed.

In order to elicit this material effectively, the Trainer needs to establish a mind-set that may at first feel out of place in the tutorial setting. It is the same state of 'split concentration' we adopt when first becoming acquainted with someone we find attractive. There is a balance of inner and outer watchfulness as we attend closely to signals coming from the other person while at the same time remaining open to our own spontaneous responses. The awareness-centred teacher cultivates this state of 'inquisitive vigilance'. Several attributes are required. First is to pay close but unobtrusive attention to the learner's minimal cues. Secondly the teacher, prompted by his own Inner Apprentice, will find his own curiosity aroused more by some cues than others. He needs to trust this curiosity and follow wherever the learner leads it, not trying to coerce the discussion to fit a pre-conceived notion of the learning agenda. Finally, there should be ever-present in the teacher's mind the questions, "What is the learner's attention on at this precise moment? What could I ask that would make him even more comprehensively aware of it?"

Forms of awareness-raising question

ARQs are designed to help a learner to access and formulate what for him are the most prominent features of his here-and-now thoughts and experience. They are elaborations of the familiar interrogatory words *'What?'*, *'Where?'*, *'When?'* and *'How?'*; but NOT (with an important exception described shortly) *'Why?'* 'Why?'-questions usually have the effect of flipping the respondent into an analytic and self-justifying answer that comes out of the memory or the imagination rather than honest immediacy. "Why?" is a question that generates fiction far more often than it prompts insight.

However, one form of 'How?'-question, *'How can you tell?'*, is in my view perennially valuable. Discussion of medical topics, albeit firmly rooted in clinical examples, easily takes flight into theory and generalisation. General Practitioners like to speculate. They tend to get nervous if left alone for too long with only the evidence of their own eyes and ears. It makes them feel like orthopaedic surgeons when they would far rather play at psychiatrists, never at a loss for an interpretation or a hypothesis. *'How can you tell?'* is a good question to recapture the fleeing attention of a Trainee scrabbling unnecessarily for an intellectual foothold and offering opinion where an account of direct experience would be more helpful.

Examples of 'What?' questions

What are you thinking?
What do you notice?
What's going through your mind?
What, if anything, strikes you about . . .?
What occurs to you at this point?
Describe what you see/think/feel.
Tell me in your own words about . . .
What did you notice about the patient at that point?
Give me some words to describe what you have noticed.
Explain to me what you mean by . . .
What direct evidence do you have for . . .?
Are you still concerned with such-and-such, or has your attention shifted to something else?

Examples of 'Where?' questions

Where is the focus of your attention at present?
Where do you think the patient's attention is?
What part of your own or the patient's body are you aware of?

Examples of 'When?' questions

When exactly did you notice . . . ?
At what point did so-and-so happen?
Tell me at what stage such-and-such a thought occurred to you.
What was it that indicated the appropriate moment for . . .?
Does such-and-such seem to vary? If so, when is it most noticeable; and when least? (And how can you tell?)
What is the sequence of events?
What happened first? What came next? And then?

Examples of 'How?' questions

How do you know that such-and-such is the case?
How can you tell?
How are you making that decision/plan?
When you do or say that, how are you deciding that it's appropriate?
How would you be able to tell whether . . .?
To what extent is such-and-such the case? Not at all? A little? A lot?
On a scale of 0 to 10, how intense is . . .?

167

How much does it vary? Between what limits?
By what process does such-and-such come about?
How sure/happy are you about this?

Indirect questions

Sentences with a question mark at the end are not the only way to pose a question. Any intervention that prompts detailed recall of past experience can function as an ARQ. So, a suggestion that prompts the memory and stimulates the imagination, or that sharpens the accuracy with which events are observed, is a legitimate way to raise awareness of data from which the Inner Apprentice can learn. For example:

Tell me what you think this issue boils down to.
Let's see if we can summarise the problem.
I see; so in a nutshell . . .
Maybe this reminds you of other similar situations.
Take your time: try and get it as clear in your own mind as you can, then tell me.
Imagine the situation as if it was on video tape: replay the tape and stop it whenever you think something significant happens. Tell me about those moments – what you notice, what you think, etc.
We've identified several aspects of the problem: prioritise them.
If there was one thing that would have affected things for the better, what would it have been?
In the given situation, if you could have had one wish granted what would you have wished?

'Why?' questions: eliciting values and beliefs

At moments when the focus of tutorial attention is on issues of factual knowledge, or on the justification for an action, or on the emotional connotations of a situation, "Why?" is not usually a particularly helpful question. "Why?" is usually answered with "Because", producing a premature switch away from immediate awareness into self-justifying theory. "Why?" tends to be interpreted as a threat to self-esteem; although cognitive dissonance may result, the associated insecurity is not always sufficiently safe to produce effective learning. Plied with too many 'Why?' questions, the learner tends to conceal ignorance or to justify false assumptions.

There is one exception. Asking 'Why?' is a very good way of raising conscious awareness of someone's values and beliefs. To be asked why we value or believe something is a seductive invitation to show how right we are. If the teacher senses that some aspect of the learner's value system is becoming an impediment to progress, a careful series of 'Why?'-questions may reveal it. The questions need to be carefully and non-judgementally phrased in order to elicit values, not facts or theory.

For example: a Trainee has prescribed ampicillin for a sore throat. "Why did you do that?", enquires the Trainer, the tone of voice implying criticism. Thus baldly asked, the question elicits a pseudo-factual answer intended to conceal ignorance and deflect challenge:

"Because it could have been a *Haemophilus* infection, and ampicillin would be appropriate."

A thankless exchange of "'Tis-'tisn't" will likely ensue.

However, the Trainer may recall that 'values are the choices we make under pressure', and might therefore phrase his question;

"Why did you choose ampicillin?", or,
"Was there some pressure on you to prescribe?", or,
"What was the deciding factor in this case?"

These variants may well be successful in eliciting value-laden responses such as:

"Because I believe in generic prescribing", or,
"Yes – I got the feeling that if I didn't the patient would only come back and see someone else", or,
"I was running late, and I felt too tired for an argument, and anyway *you* do it sometimes too!"

Clearly discernible in these latter answers are value-rich cues that, if pursued with sensitive tenacity, may well lead the tutorial to a highly-charged point of kairos.

Other forms of the value-eliciting "Why?" might be:

"What was the underlying reason for . . .?";
"What made you opt for . . . ?";
"Why does . . . seem preferable?";
"Why not consider . . .?"
"What was it about this that made you think/feel/say . . .?";
"What principles are involved here?";
"What would your opinion be about . . .?"
"Why do you make . . . a priority?".

Timing, pacing and follow-through

In an ideal and over-simplified world, where learners were transparently honest and insatiably thirsty for knowledge and their teachers supremely skilful and perceptive, ARQs should be capable of refining any tutorial discussion from low-key generalities to a point of kairos with remorseless inevitability. But human attention is not so robotic. Both learner and teacher are fatiguable. Both have blind spots and no-go areas which are deferred items on the day's educational agenda. The 'butterfly flutter' described earlier – brief excursions into apparently irrelevant side-issues – is one outward sign of the limited time-span for which an awareness-centred approach can be sustained. Another indication is the way attention spontaneously oscillates between being inner-directed and outer-directed, as described in the section on 'Rhythmicity' in Chapter 5, pages 108–113, Figures 5.2 and 5.3. The learner's attention is directed unconsciously by processes I have called the 'Inner Apprentice', and these mechanisms are ultimately trustworthy. However, most people experience a need at frequent intervals to take 'time out' for their conscious intellects to catch up with and take stock of their unconsciously-acquired learning increments. Awareness-centred learning therefore needs to alternate with periods of reflection and conscious integration.

How is this cyclical pattern of awareness-raising alternating with reflection to be paced? My personal view is that awareness-centred teaching should predominate as long as the learner remains genuinely absorbed and interested in what his here-and-now attention can reveal. It is not usually difficult for the observant teacher to recognise from the learner's minimal cues whether or not he is 'genuinely absorbed' in retrieving and recounting direct sensory experience. In particular there will be frequent signs of internal search – physical stillness accompanied by upwards or downwards shifts of gaze, or by defocussing of the eyes. Readiness to shift from awareness to analysis mode may be signalled by restlessness, by a reduction in internal search, and by unresponsiveness to ARQs.

When, during an awareness-centred phase of discussion, the learner's interest shows signs of flagging, it may be timely for the teacher to assist the disengagement by adopting a consciously reflective or analytic style. For instance he may ask, "What have you learned from this? What lessons will you take away? What will you do differently in future? Let's summarise what we've established so far." Before long the period of analysis induced by this switch will itself in turn begin to pall and feel sterile. The options then exist either of returning to an awareness-centred mode of enquiry, or of deciding that "that's enough for today". The choice depends on whether or not a significant point of kairos has been attained; if not, another round of awareness-raising and reflection might be in order.

Figure 8.1 charts the progress of a learner's attention as the tutorial's cyclical process carries it towards the kairotic moment when real learning is set to occur.

Whether formal set-piece tutorial or opportunistic 'hot topic' discussion, a session of teaching and learning usually starts at a fairly superficial level. Both parties tend by tacit agreement initially to confine themselves to pleasantries, generalities and superficialities: or, if depth is attempted, it is a comfortable and well-rehearsed depth. From these early omnipotential exchanges there soon emerges an initial focus of attention which both agree to examine more closely. The learner's opening gambit, and particularly any associated curtain-raisers, provide useful cues. (And this book's contention is that, if the teacher will resist the inclination to direct this early focussing and instead can allow his interventions to be shaped by the learner's minimal cues, the learner's Inner Apprentice will draw his own attention to a focus in which the pertinent lesson is already latent.)

Watchful for minimal cues of cognitive dissonance in the learner, such as speech censoring, speech turbulence or displacement activities, the teacher shifts into a more awareness-raising style of facilitation. The learner's attention will be seen to become progressively more inner-directed, as evidenced by changes in gaze, changes in vocal tone and delivery, increase in personalised 'I'-statements, and perhaps the unex-pected value-laden phrase or micro-emotion. ARQs are now used to help the learner gain maximal access to his stream of awareness undistracted by attempts to 'make sense of it'. To notice and to explore are sufficient. This is the stage of absorption, when the insecurity of mounting cognitive dissonance is kept safe by the teacher's unobtrusive and non-judgemental encouragement.

Before long, usually within a few minutes, introspection has gone as far as for the moment it seems safe to do so, and the learner's attention will spontaneously disengage and become outer-directed again. There may be an abrupt change of posture, tone of voice or subject matter; vocabulary becomes less personal, more abstract and conceptual; humour or appar-ent irrelevancies may occur, temporarily dispelling internal tensions. The teacher needs to recognise this moment of disengagement, for to persist now with an awareness-raising approach will be unrewarding or even alienating. Both now stand back, and in discussion review and reflect upon whatever thoughts have just emerged. This is the appropriate time

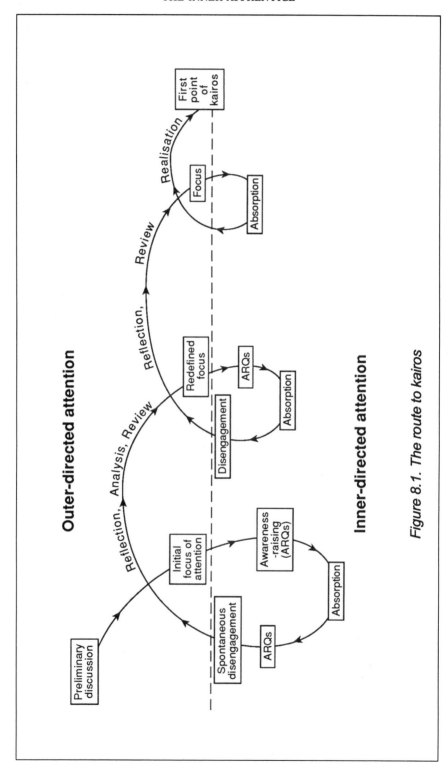

Figure 8.1. The route to kairos

for the teacher to offer analysis, criticism, interpretation, advice, factual input, summarising, hypothesising and forward planning. The offer should be tempered with reticence, however; the teacher may believe he can 'see what's needed' well before the learner achieves a similar clarity. What to the teacher seems the obvious lesson may well, for the learner, not yet be the kairotic one.

From this 'reflection phase' a new redefined focus of attention may emerge, a step or two nearer to the session's first point of kairos. As this secondary focus is addressed the learner's attention begins to turn inwards again, and the cycle of awareness-raising, absorption, disengagement and review can be repeated. By this iterative process the learner's perspicacity is progressively sharpened, until, at the point of kairos, the most pressing educational need can be discerned starkly yet safely. Several cycles of focus/awareness-raising/absorption/disengagement/review may be needed to carry the tide of educational opportunity from what *might* be learned to the kairotic *must*.

An example of these principles at work in a tutorial might help. The dialogue is fictitious and abbreviated; the dilemma universal.

Case illustration

> *Trainer:* I see you had a night visit to the Hooligans last night. Would you like to tell me about it?
>
> *Trainee:* *(with a snort)* Don't you find there are some night calls you just can't get back to sleep afterwards? ... Anyway, this was the four-year-old who'd got a cold. When I got there I just gave the usual advice.

There is an immediate incongruity between the straightforward triviality of the Trainee's opening gambit ("four-year-old, cold, advice") and the latent anger and resentment in the curtain-raising snort and remark about disturbed sleep. This incongruity indicates significant cognitive dissonance, alerting us to a potential learning need and suggesting an initial focus for tutorial attention.

> *Trainer:* It sounds as if we can take the clinical bits for granted. How about the not getting back to sleep?
>
> *Trainee:* I think there was just too much adrenalin flowing. Have you got any suggestions? Would you have not made a visit, and dealt with it on the telephone?

Even if he had suggestions, it would be premature for the Trainer to proffer them yet. The Trainee's Inner Apprentice has clearly also registered the same initial focus, namely, dealing with the feelings aroused by clinically inappropriate night calls. So far, however, the fine detail of the problem has not been made fully conscious, nor the associated knowledge gap rendered explicit. The Trainer shifts into awareness-raising mode.

Trainer: How do you mean, adrenalin?

Trainee: Well, I was all churned up.

The 'adrenalin' remark and the expression 'churned up' are, respectively, a non sequitur and an imprecision indicating significant speech censoring. The speaker anticipates that acknowledging a deficit in his coping skills may pose some threat to his self-esteem, and the resulting cognitive dissonance causes him to oversimplify and prevaricate.

Trainer: What kind of churned up?

Trainee: A mixture: irritation mostly, and feeling I shouldn't have to be at people's beck and call for trivia like that. Inexperience, maybe, helplessness.

Trainer: What's the strongest feeling that's stayed with you?

Trainee: Irritation. Yes, definitely irritation!

The Trainer can 'hear' the last exclamation mark in the pitch and animation of the Trainee's voice, and notices that the eyes are briefly lowered in internal search and the head nods briefly in emphasis. To ask "Why were you irritated?" at this stage begs the self-justifying answer "Anyone would be, to be got out of bed just for a cold!" Instead the Trainer maintains the awareness-raising line:

Trainer: Tell me what was said.

Trainee: Well Mrs Hooligan demanded a call, and I satisfied myself it was just a cold the child had, but she insisted, so I gritted my teeth and . . .

Trainer: Slow down, slow down. Pretend there was a video camera recording the conversation. Rewind the video, replay it in your mind's eye, and see if you can recall exactly what was said.

Trainee: Word for word?

Trainer: Word for word.

Prolonged internal search ensues as the Trainee tries to recall specific detail; the stilted quality of the account now indicates a genuine effort to retell the conversation 'as it happened'. Absence of eye contact indicates that his attention has now become inner-directed. This is the stage of absorption, the Trainee being fully engrossed in calling up the detailed memory of his recent experience into full awareness. We pick up the dialogue shortly afterwards.

Trainee: . . . 'Try some paracetamol', then she said 'Are you coming or aren't you?', and I said 'Oh all right' . . .

Trainer: Calmly, like that? No? How, then?

Trainee: 'OH ALL RIGHT!' But I was feeling pretty cross by then.

Trainer: I'm sure you were. When precisely did you start to feel cross? What was it that pressed the button?

Trainee: It wasn't when Mrs H. first said she wanted a visit; it was the 'Are you coming or aren't you?'

Trainer: What did you feel like saying to her at that moment?

This last is a highly challenging question, and the Trainee is unsettled by realising what he might reveal in his reply. His attention disengages from the narrative, he resumes eye contact, smiles, perhaps breathes deeply, and there is a change in his vocal range.

Trainee: Yes, well! . . . But then I remembered what we were saying about the child as presenting symptom, and I wondered whether there might be some underlying marital problem.

Trainer: Or maybe a history of serious illness either in this child or one of her others.

Trainee: Anyway, getting up at night's all part of the job, isn't it?"

The reflection, analysis and review phase is now well established, and may continue for a while on familiar lines. The first cycle of awareness-raising reaches a tentative and only temporary conclusion.

> *Trainee:*   . . . and yes, I did remember the night visit claim form. *(Pause)* It's just that I feel I kind of let myself down by letting her get to me.

With this value-laden phrase the Trainee signals readiness to redirect attention inwards, and so a second cycle of awareness-raising questioning is appropriate. The focus has now become more sharply defined: the problem is not simply that the Trainee was annoyed, but that he has some uncomfortable feelings about the possible significance of his anger. Before accepting this refined version as the secondary focus, the Trainer needs to be sure that this aspect of the case is also of strong here-and-now interest to the Trainee.

> *Trainer:*   It seems there are two issues. One is how Mrs H. managed to provoke you, and the other is whether or not you should feel badly about your reaction. Which seems to you to be more important now?
>
> *Trainee:*   My reaction. I mean, a good doctor should be able to take this sort of thing in his stride, shouldn't he, and deal with an unnecessary night visit without getting so upset?

With this "*shouldn't he?*" the Trainee reveals a limiting belief system which (on this occasion at least) is operating against the interests of his peace of mind. In this situation a 'Why?'-question is appropriate to elicit the underlying values. We are now into the awareness-raising phase of the second cycle, the second surge of the tutorial tide.

> *Trainer:*   You reckon only bad doctors get upset, is that right? Why do you take that view?
>
> *Trainee:*   I just think it's unprofessional not to be able to control one's reactions. I admire doctors who don't let this sort of situation upset them.
>
> *Trainer:*   *(remembering that values are the choices we make under pressure, and so imposing some pressure)* If there are such doctors, why should you admire them? Why should you not envy them their equanimity? Or criticise them for being out of touch with their feelings?
>
> *Trainee:*   Because – I don't know; it's just the way I am.

This last exchange is an extremely rapid cycle of awareness-raising, absorption, disengaging and review. Pursued with 'Why?'-questions, the Trainee's belief about how he 'should' react is revealed as only one of several tenable positions, and a possibly maladaptive one at that. A moment of Socratic *aporia* is reached: *"Because – I don't know!"*. The Trainee realises that further heart-searching will still leave his problem unresolved, and so his attention disengages. The remark *"it's just the way I am"* represents an abbreviated review phase, leading discussion to a second possible end-point of this second cycle of awareness-raising.

However, finding himself and his values on shifting sands the Trainee's feelings of cognitive dissonance will not be adequately dispelled by so simplistic a conclusion. It would be easy to rescue him with a supportive remark such as "Even professionals are made out of mortal flesh and blood", but by staying in awareness-raising mode the Trainer allows the Trainee's Inner Apprentice a chance to discover its own solution. A pause ensues, perhaps punctuated with inappropriate humour or fidgeting, during which signs of internal search are visible. When it ends, the Trainer can try to elicit a third focus of attention.

Trainer: What was going through your mind just then?

Trainee: I was thinking, when Mrs Hooligan said was I coming or wasn't I, what I felt like telling her was, 'Look, it's late, and I'm tired, and I know I've got to come out, but don't expect me to be pleased about it, and don't just take me for granted!' Of course I wouldn't dream of coming out with all that, but that's what kept going round in my head, and it stopped me getting back to sleep.

Vestiges of emotion are audible at this point in the Trainee's voice, indicating that the issue is still current and that a third cycle of awareness-raising, this time focussing explicitly on learning needs, is therefore appropriate.

Trainer: In a situation like this, what do you wish you could do that would make you feel better?

Trainee: I'd like to be able to get rid of my angry feelings without being unsympathetic to the patient.

Trainer: Let's see if we can be a little more specific. How would you like to behave while you're actually on the phone to Mrs Hooligan?

Trainee:	Stay calm and polite; not get riled; just take the details. I don't usually have a problem doing that, at the time. It's while I'm driving to the house that I feel worst.
Trainer:	So what you'd like to be able to do instead is . . .?
Trainee:	Get it out of my system before I reach the patient. So that I'm clear-minded by the time I'm there.
Trainer:	And do you have any ways of achieving that?
Trainee:	No, apart from muttering to myself. And that obviously doesn't work, or I wouldn't still be churned up when I get back home.
Trainer:	Take a moment to think about this; see if you can summarize as clearly as you can what new skills or resources this episode has shown you that you need.
Trainee:	Okay. *(Pause: then, hesitantly)* I could do with . . . *(More internal search: now definitely and with confidence)* What I need are some ways to off-load my own negative feelings harmlessly or even constructively.

Kairos. The Trainee's systematic exploration of what lay behind his initial curtain-raising remark has highlighted an important educational need with an almost desperate clarity. Now, even if a solution proves elusive, the problem is well-posed and the Trainee hungry for help. Now, and only now, is whatever assistance the Trainer can provide likely to be truly welcomed. He might suggest playing loud music in the car, or joining a Balint group, or learning a stress management technique such as Autogenic Training. The two of them might role-play some assertiveness techniques in the name of what is euphemistically termed 'modifying the patient's help-seeking behaviour'. My point is, once the nub of the Trainee's problem has been accurately elicited through his own introspection, devising the 'best available solution' is not so difficult. The right problem is easier to solve than the wrong one, and the right lesson easier to learn than the wrong.

(For what it's worth, my current personal favourite solution to the 'how not to get cross' problem is as follows. When you want to be angry, only getting angry will help. You need to do some 'being angry' behaviour. But it doesn't have to be directed at the real target. Oneself will do. Try berating yourself on the way to see the patient: "Call yourself a doctor? My cat's got more sympathy! Here you are, well paid, driving a nice car, doing no more than the job you're trained for, and you have the nerve to complain when . . ." Within half a minute irritation dissolves as the stupidity of such a soliloquy melts into laughter.)

Mutative information

At the point of kairos, the learner is maximally receptive to mutative (change-producing and growth-enhancing) information which can fill the knowledge gap newly and compellingly perceived. For maximum effectiveness mutative information needs to be:

- *congruent with the learner's existing values and beliefs*, so that new ideas are in line with the learner's personal sense of mission as he or she currently perceives it;
- *non-judgementally presented*, so that suggestions can be incorporated without traumatising the learner's self-esteem and arousing fresh cognitive dissonance;
- *tailored to the specific situation* that engendered the need, so that the benefits of the new learning can be clearly envisioned;
- *carefully observed as it impacts* on the learner, so that by detecting minimal cues of acceptance or rejection the teacher can best phrase, pace and structure his intervention.

On how to decide what information is mutative in the given circumstances, and on how it might be presented, I propose to say nothing. Given the high degree of concentration and concern for the other person produced in the teacher by the process of awareness-raising, the teacher will find that he spontaneously intervenes with appropriate skill and insight when a point of kairos is reached. All necessary knowledge, experience and sensitivity are pre-resident in the teacher; his own training and the motivation that have led him to teach will guarantee that. The state of mind that accompanies the pupil to a kairotic insight is the same state of mind that releases the teacher's helpfulness when it is needed. On the moment-by-moment time-scale we are considering, it is enough for the teacher to recognise the various minimal cues, to be guided by them in the process of awareness-raising and to follow them to a point of kairos, and then – to respond however comes naturally.

Eavesdropping on our fictitious tutorial a little later on, we might hear:

Trainer: . . . so, having chuntered away at yourself as you drive to the Hooligans, the last thing a good doctor does before ringing the doorbell is . . .

Trainee:	. . . tell myself that some skilful patient education now will save me aggravation in the future.
Trainer:	So, after you've examined the child and advised accordingly, you'll say . . .?
Trainee:	I'll say, 'Before I go, Mrs Hooligan, there's something else I want to explain to you. I think you knew it was just a cold that Buster had, so another time . . .
Trainer:	Excellent. I don't suppose you'll find it any easier than the rest of us to put good intentions into action, but what you've planned there is certainly the counsel of perfection for future occasions.

Obstacles to effective awareness-raising

Reduced to its simplest, awareness-centred teaching requires of the teacher that a higher than usual proportion of his attention be directed outwardly onto minimal cues emitted by the learner, and less of it inwardly trying to work out 'what ought to be taught'. We have seen how a subliminal awareness of what needs to be learned is pre-resident in the learner; but the cues signalling those needs have first to be noticed and secondly to be trusted. The awareness-centred teacher sets greater store on noticing than on telling. To a far greater extent than we usually allow, learning *is* noticing; and the process of assisting the learner to notice *is* the process of teaching, not just the prelude to it.

Unfortunately most of us medical teachers have been indoctrinated with the conventional curriculum-based educational cycle of objectives, strategies and assessment – 'plan, tell, test'. 'Telling' is our default mode; the alternative of 'active noticing' does not come easily. Some puritan part of us seems to believe that 'proper' education should be hard work, and that 'good' teaching should be a telling military campaign against native ignorance. So we have something of a trust problem. It feels like a betrayal of responsibility to entrust a measure of the teacher's customary role of guiding, pacing and directing to the learner's intrinsic learning mechanisms – the Inner Apprentice. Yet without such trust we seem destined to stay locked in an almost feudal relationship of teller and told, leader and led.

To be thought an expert is a flattering, seductive and easily addictive notion. And the unfortunate word 'Trainee' has associations of passivity and inferiority, reinforcing an easy tendency for Trainer and Trainee to lapse into a relationship, however benevolent and amicable, where the expertise of the one is complemented by subservience in the other. While this dynamic may be comfortable overall, even helpful, as a way of doing moment-by-moment teaching it has its limitations. It allows a mirage to form, a fallacy that there is such a thing as 'quick fix education'. Because General Practice is 'the art so long to learn', and because a year is so short an apprenticeship, we feel under great pressure of time to cover enormous tracts of learning at a breathless pace. But it is time to question whether curriculum-based methodology is really the pair of seven-league boots we thought we needed.

A Trainee once made me a gift of a pad of novelty stick-on notes; and for a while the messages I left him bore the printed legend 'From the desk of God'. Then he started leaving *me* notes, taken from a companion pad of his own. They were headed 'Trust me – I'm an expert'.

One of the epigrams to this chapter – 'Learn to recognize beginnings' – is from *The Tao of Leadership* [4], John Heider's updating of the ancient laid-back wisdom about managing human resources as expounded by the Chinese sage Lao Tzu. The following extract is taken from a section called 'The Beginning, the Middle, and the End'.

> Learn to recognize beginnings. At birth, events are relatively easy to manage. Slight interventions shape and guide easily . . . The greatest danger lies in disrupting the emerging process by using too much force. . .
>
> Once an event is fully energized and formed, stand back as much as possible. Needless interventions will only confuse or block what is happening. Especially do not try to make an event conform to any predetermined plan or model.
>
> Many leaders spoil the work just as it nears completion. They get eager. They get invested in certain outcomes. They become anxious and make mistakes. This is a time for care and consciousness. Don't do too much. Don't be too helpful. Don't worry about getting credit for having done something.
>
> Because the wise leader has no expectations, no outcome can be called a failure. Paying attention, allowing a natural unfolding, and standing back most of the time, the leader sees the event arrive at a satisfactory conclusion.
>
> [op. cit. p. 127]

Chapter 9
The Inner Curriculum

In completing one discovery we never fail to get an imperfect knowledge of others of which we could have no idea before, so that we cannot solve one doubt without creating several new ones.

Joseph Priestley,
Experiments and Observations
on Different Kinds of Air, 1775–86

The inner-directed analysis in previous chapters has left the tutorial process anatomised. We might wonder whether the fragments can ever reconstitute themselves into the living and purposive experience of a professional apprenticeship.

It is as if we were to find ourselves in the Pointillists room of an art gallery, standing just eighteen inches away from Seurat's painting *La Baignade*. From close up our field of view is filled with discrete dabs of colour; each dot vibrant and interesting enough in its way, we suppose, but arbitrary, lacking relationship and purpose. We see no frame, no edges, no outlines, no design – until we step back. Then the dots meld into shapes, figures, events, meaning, an image complete and evocative, the seemingly random revealed as the truly accomplished. Ah, we think; the artist knew what he was about. Jehovah-like he held the completed image in his mind's eye as he dabbed and dotted. He knew what dots of what colour would eventually summate to his inner vision. And then, a disturbing thought. What if it wasn't *the artist* who knew what dot needed to go where? What if it was *the image* that knew? What if *the dots knew* the picture they were part of, and somehow ordered their own disposition? What if Seurat was merely the channel through which the dots could proclaim, "We know the whole whereof we are parts"? Many an artist will tell you, "It was the picture directed the brush"; and a novelist, "The characters dictated their own story" . . .

182

I hope by now the reader may allow that it is possible, even desirable, to base and pace an individual teaching session on the promptings of the learner's Inner Apprentice, i.e. a preconscious learning mechanism that knows what it needs to learn, and that signals its need as the recognisable cues of cognitive dissonance. Teaching proceeds by raising non-judgemental awareness of these cues to the kairotic point where learning becomes inevitable. But it is far from self-evident that we can place the same reliance on the learner's internally-dictated agenda when it comes to programming the more sustained educational trajectory of a Traineeship lasting many months. It is one thing to credit the Inner Apprentice with creating learning opportunities in the immediate context of a single tutorial. But there is no reason to suppose it can also function on the larger canvas and the longer time-scale. Or can it? Is it dotty to suppose that there might indeed be an Inner Curriculum, capable of reliably structuring its own optimum syllabus in appropriate sequence, with rigour and sensitivity, paying due attention both to blind spots and to the loftiest aspirations of self-fulfilment?

My thesis to this point has been that teaching is largely a matter of seeing to it that an appropriate awareness of the learner's subliminal curiosity gets raised, safely yet resolutely. In this chapter we shall see whether this principle, applied on the larger scale, reveals an Inner Curriculum, in which issues of value and belief, mission and motivation are addressed – not because a teacher wills it but because that is the intrinsic nature of the Inner Apprentice. Are there ways of raising non-judgemental awareness of values and motivation? And what happens if we do?

Epiphanies

I think most teachers will recognise this phenomenon: events unpredictably confront a Trainee with a particularly complex and daunting problem, a challenge to his competence so threatening that he doubts his ability to cope with it. But in fact he is more ready than he had supposed. Without his realising it, prior learning has established all necessary component skills like a trail of stacked up dominoes awaiting the single nudge that will send them cascading into a new stability. And though for the Trainee the experience at the time may be stressful, and he may feel as much out of control as the toppling dominoes, there remains ever afterwards an abiding sense that something significant has happened, some Rubicon been crossed, some new maturity acquired. Had the same challenge been faced at an earlier stage it might have proved overwhelming; and if later, commonplace. But from time to time in the trajectory of learning there are critical periods when the learner is primed for a particular breakthrough. Competence takes a sudden stride forward which can never be reversed. It is as if some part of the learner knew the lesson that was needed, and seized – created? – the opportunity for it. The experience is usually attended by strong emotion as 'the scales fall from one's eyes' – relief or pleasure, renewed motivational energy, even tears. Saint Paul on the road to Damascus is perhaps the most famous example of this phenomenon, which I'll call an *epiphany*. Instances abound in vocational training, less dramatic but nonetheless important to the individual, of the epiphany principle:

When the pupil is ready, the lesson appears.

Case illustration

Six months into her Traineeship Rebecca is doing well. She is well liked by colleagues and patients. Her medical knowledge is sound, and she has managed to shift her clinical thinking from the systematic approach of hospital medicine to the hypothesis-testing of general practice without too much difficulty. Recently she has become interested in the dynamics of the doctor–patient relationship, and has read various texts on the consultation process. At their last formal tutorial, she and her Trainer discussed Balint's ideas on the way the doctor's own feelings can function therapeutically as pointers to the patient's emotional state.

It is Rebecca's day on call. In the morning she saw six-month-old Rees Morton, who had a cold. It was clearly just a cold, and she spent some time explaining how antibiotics were not needed and discussing how Rees' mother sometimes felt inadequate, her own parents living many miles away. It is now nine o'clock in the evening, and Rebecca's phone rings. "Get round here quick!" shrieks a man who proves to be Rees' father. "The baby's dead."

And so he is; a cot death. At the house Rebecca confirms death, contacts the appropriate officials, pays sympathetic attention to the parents' grief. It is a struggle for her to maintain any semblance of professionalism; the truth is that she too is engulfed in a morass of misery. Guilt, panic, sorrow and remorse alternate with the wish to justify herself to the distraught parents. Rebecca's turmoil of self-reproach is a good deal more anguished than mere cognitive dissonance. "It was just a cold; I couldn't have known; it's not my fault!" is what she doesn't say. She torments herself with accusatory visions of the Coroner's court, litigation, whispers and pointing fingers. The baby's father approaches her, arm outstretched, hand up-raised. For a moment she thinks he is about to strike her in a fury she feels she well deserves.

But no; Huw Morton draws her towards him, until each head rests on the other's shoulder. Hugging her he mutters, "You must feel terrible." Thus acknowledged, Rebecca bursts into unsuppressable tears as she realises he sees her not as 'the doctor who let us down' but as a fellow victim of life's wretched and arbitrary unfairness. Acceptance of her human frailty and fallibility dynamites its way into her professional persona, and will abide there forever.

The first domino has fallen; and for the remainder of that evening and for some time to come Rebecca's mind is preoccupied with the clatter as others she had thought secure continue to topple. The management of minor illness in infants; various theories of cot death; the role of support groups; the stages of the grieving process; the management of emotional catharsis; awareness of the doctor's own feelings – all the dominoes were stacked up independently in Rebecca's store of knowledge before Mrs Morton ever consulted. Now she *knows* these things in a different and more integrated way. With Rees' death they have fallen into place in a concatenation of learning that will in fact be mostly complete by the time she next sees her Trainer. He will no doubt help her see that her present distress is what the old apprentice-masters used to call 'the craft entering the body'. Together they will make bearable sense of a lesson all vocational journeymen learn before they graduate: we-the-professional and we-the-person are running a race over hurdles, and in real life either can win.

Had these events occurred earlier or later in the trajectory of her Trainee-ship Rebecca would probably have learned different things from them. Had she been less aware of the impact of the doctor's own feelings on the therapeutic process, or of how impossible it is to predict the course of every illness at its unformed outset, it is likely she would have found herself regressing into the defensive style of practice she learned in hospital, where the little white-coated inner voice constantly whispers in the junior doctor's ear, "Cover your butt, and don't get involved." Conversely, had she been in practice rather longer her soft shell might have become case-hardened into a carapace of apparent nonchalance, and the lesson that her own spontaneous feelings are trustworthy might have been lost to her. As it is, there is a fair chance that Rebecca, when her initial agitation subsides, will have matured significantly. She will be more aware of her own limitations; better equipped to manage uncertainty; perhaps she will be motivated to join a Balint group, or go on to some formal counselling training.

When the pupil is ready, the lesson appears: the readiness endows chance events with serendipity. It is the learner's internal agenda that renders an opportunity timely. Learning on the 'epiphany' scale of Rebecca's may occur relatively infrequently, but on a few occasions in a Traineeship we have the sense that the educational agenda has abruptly moved on to a new plateau. The learning curve is not smooth, neither does it meander aimlessly. It consists of sudden purposive increments alternating with apparent pauses, while the Inner Apprentice invisibly incorporates new knowledge and silently establishes its next learning agenda. The learner ascends step-wise a succession of levels, a succession of vantage points, arranged in tiers. In other words, the sequence of educational issues to which the learner's attention finds itself drawn as time goes by – the inner curriculum – forms a hierarchy.

THE INNER CURRICULUM

Maslow's hierarchy of needs

Wie ihr es immer dreht und wie ihr's immer schiebt
Erst kommt das Fressen, dann kommt die Moral.
(No matter how you turn or twist it,
Food comes first, morals later on.)

Ballad – *"What keeps a man alive?"*,
from Bertolt Brecht's libretto to Kurt Weill's
The Threepenny Opera, 1928

As we begin to discern some structure in the array of educational issues, and to recognise that prioritizing and sequencing are important, we might see what can be learned from Abraham Maslow's original work on the hierarchical arrangement of human needs [1]. Maslow made extensive studies of how it comes about that some fortunate individuals seem to fulfil all their native potential, while others appear fated to remain under-fulfilled and blocked. He concluded that if we list all the various needs and motivations that people from time to time experience we can arrange them pyramid-wise in the form of a hierarchy. At the base are the most fundamental and essential needs, those which if unsatisfied jeopardise our very survival. Above these, arranged like the tiers on a wedding cake, come layers of need which are progressively more optional, more discretionary.

Figure 9.1 displays Maslow's 'map' of human motivation. In this model, human needs are fulfilled from the bottom upwards. We are predominantly driven by the lowest level of unmet need. Once our needs at one level are substantially met, motivational energy becomes automatically redirected towards satisfying needs at the next level up. These in turn preoccupy us until their attainment releases an awareness of, and a quest for fulfilment of, goals at yet higher levels in the hierarchy.

At the bottom of the hierarchy physiological needs are the most pressing: requirements for air and food, biochemical normality, sleep and sexual relief. When felt, these take precedence over everything else. These needs being satisfied, we are next impelled to create a safe physical environment for ourselves, followed by what Maslow called a need for 'belongingness' – a safe and supportive emotional and psychological network. Once we feel we truly 'belong' somewhere, we look next for the appreciation and esteem of other people, first those near to us then others more remote. When we know we are respected by other people we internalise this esteem and experience a sense of *self*-esteem, of *self*-respect, thereby feeling ourselves to have been granted permission to strive after the full expression of whatever potential resides within us.

Maslow's researches help us understand why some things are more important than others, some needs more pressing, some priorities more immediate. They explain why, for instance, one cannot easily discuss philosophy with a full bladder, chair a committee on an empty stomach, or make love in the pouring rain. Maslow enables us to predict, in general terms at least, which of two simultaneous drives will prevail – the one lower in the hierarchy. He indicates what we should do if one level of aspiration seems to remain out of reach – concentrate on gratifying any unmet needs at the next level down. Once these are adequately addressed an impulse to pursue higher-order goals will be released without forcing.

Maslow's account, like all models when they attempt to reduce human complexity to manageable proportions, is an over-simplification. The sceptic will rightly remind us that no need is ever completely and permanently satiated; that we frequently have to settle for 'good enough to be going on with', and are often none the worse for that; that some needs can be sublimated or leap-frogged, or their gratification delayed; that it is possible to live a whole lifetime with permanent gaps at all levels of need and still function effectively. Yet to my mind Maslow's insights survive these qualifications. Human development, and the needs and

SELF–ACTUALIZATION NEEDS

Realization of innate potential
Self-fulfilment
Self-expression

Self-esteem
Self-respect
Self-confidence

ESTEEM NEEDS

Esteem
Status
Approval
Appreciation
Recognition

'BELONGINGNESS' NEEDS

Love
Intimacy
Affection
Someone to confide in
Friendship
Company
Acknowledgement

SAFETY NEEDS

Boundaries
Predictability
Stability
Warmth and shelter
Security
Roots
Freedom from fear and anxiety

PHYSIOLOGICAL NEEDS

Sex
Sleep
Normal physiological parameters
Food and drink
Oxygen

Figure 9.1 Hierarchy of human needs, after Maslow

motivations that drive it, is not an inflexible sequence. But an evolutionary sequence it nonetheless is. Human motivational growth unfolds
along a steady trajectory of emphasis that defies the random vicissitudes of
circumstance. The trajectory may be thrown off course, aborted and
distorted, its end-point limited by unlucky accidents of fate or inheritance.
Nevertheless the unfolding of motivational stages is ordered according to
a pre-resident internal programme; that is to say, while we look to the
environment to supply the means of satisfying each felt need in turn,
external pressure is not required – indeed, is not able – to compel the
direction or arbitrarily inflate the strength of our urges. Direction and
magnitude come from within. They stem from the interaction of past
experience and the innate sequence of needs described by Maslow.
Exhortation generates little in the way of aspirational energy: prior
satisfaction of subordinate needs does.

The hierarchy of educational imperatives

It requires but a short intuitive leap to wonder whether Maslow's
'intrinsic hierarchy' principle can usefully be transferred into other areas
of human endeavour, in particular that of vocational education. Clearly,
given all that has gone before, I shall contend that it can. It seems to me
that an educational trajectory can be mapped in this hierarchical way,
and that such a map furnishes a description of every learner's intrinsic
learning programme – the Inner Curriculum.

Some Traineeships, particularly the more curriculum-dominated ones,
seem to proceed on a 'bingo card' principle, systematically ticking off
various topics and objectives in fairly random order until play ends after
the twelve allotted months. What can easily be lost in this approach is,
first, a sensitivity to the educational dynamics operating on a larger-than-
piecemeal timescale, and secondly an appreciation of how important it is
for the teacher to work in harmony with fluctuations in the learner's own
readiness. A Traineeship, like a medieval apprenticeship, is a long enough
period of personal involvement for us to speak of its trajectory – its arising,
unfolding, achieving and ending. Traineeships, like life cycles, go through
the equivalents of birth, growth, adolescence, maturity, ageing and
bereavement. Like love affairs they have phases of meeting, courtship,
intimacy, tiffs and reconciliations, pride and disappointment, euphoria
and grief.

Figure 9.2 is an attempt to translate Maslow's principles into an
educational context. Other teachers must be the judges of its value and
accuracy; but it seems to be a 'good enough' first draft of the curriculum
the Inner Apprentice works to. In an ideal world the trajectory of a

AUTONOMY
>   Takes responsibility for own continuing education
>   Successfully negotiates transition from Trainee to Principal
>   Finds and maintains ways to enhance job satisfaction
>   Discovers, chooses and pursues own interests
>   Sense of overall purpose, worth and direction

SELF-ESTEEM
>   Feels comfortable with, not oppressed by, Trainee role
>   Can use self in consultations: 'Balint-wise'
>   Comfortable balance between private and professional life
>   Not addicted to an idealised 'doctor' role
>   Tolerates uncertainty, inadequacy, and occasional failure
>   Negotiates and organises own educational programme
>   Takes pride in keeping clinically well-informed and up-to-date
>   Knows own strengths and limitations
>   Can advise, challenge, and constructively criticise Trainer
>   Aware of transference issues in Trainer/Trainee relationship

RECOGNITION
>   Hungry for new ideas and experiences
>   Aware of, and willing to address, own needs and motivations
>   Interested in 'softer' topics, e.g. hidden agenda, consultation skills, doctor/patient relationship
>   Can accept criticism and praise
>   Attracts a personal following of patients
>   Confidence not dependent on Trainer's approval

CONFIDENCE
>   Accepted by, and contributes to, primary health care team
>   Involves other team members appropriately
>   Willing to take responsibility: can 'hold' situations
>   Makes and manages psychological and social diagnoses
>   Recognises and rectifies clinical blind-spots
>   Deals competently with minor illness and atypical presentations
>   'Bonding' with Trainer

SAFETY
>   Availability of Trainer's help and support
>   Able and willing to ask for help
>   Availability of books and information resources
>   Competent in dealing with urgent and straightforward physical illness
>   Basic clinical knowledge and skills

SURVIVAL
>   Timetable; protected time
>   Own room, desk, equipment
>   Working knowledge of prescriptions, certificates, forms
>   Local geography, medical facilities, services, telephone numbers
>   Knowledge of surgery arrangements, names of staff
>   Free from non-professional worries, e.g. health, money, personal

Figure 9.2 Hierarchy of educational imperatives -
'The Inner Curriculum'

Traineeship would be a steady upward journey from the bottom 'Survival' level to 'Autonomy' at the top. As in the Maslow original, at any given stage of his or her education the learner is chiefly preoccupied with the lowest level of unaddressed business. The learner's current level of attainment in the hierarchy defines what particular aspect of a given clinical problem will be singled out for consideration out of all its possible challenges.

'Survival' issues

'Physiological' needs were in Maslow's terms the most imperative, prolonged frustration of them being unsurvivable. They have an educational equivalent insofar as some basic physical and informational conditions have to be established and maintained before the metabolic processes of training can occur. New Trainees must rapidly become familiar with the day-to-day arrangements of the practice and the names and roles of its personnel. They will feel at sea without a working knowledge of the geography of the practice area, its landmarks and its key medical facilities such as hospitals, pharmacies, clinics, and their access arrangements including telephone numbers. Incoming Trainees are usually daunted by the paper-work of General Practice, and feel themselves to be floundering unless quickly given guidance in writing prescriptions, issuing certificates and filling in the various forms essential to the practice's smooth running. Many training practices provide this information in the form of a hand-book.

Trainees newly implanting in the womb of a training practice need to establish a safe zone for themselves, some fixed points of familiarity amid the turbulence. Often this need is symbolically met by buying their own 'black bag' and diagnostic equipment. It seems important for a new Trainee to be given his or her own room, together with permission to personalise it. The daily and weekly timetable, including periods of protected time for teaching or study, needs to be established, not merely for its utility value but also for the sense of 'firm ground beneath the feet' it conveys.

All this is familiar territory for Trainers. Familiarity, however, carries the danger of taking such basic educational pre-requisites for granted. Assumptions are easily made, plans compromised and protected time eroded. Because these 'survival' issues are so basic Trainees may not like to confess the need to re-visit them. For educational life to flourish both Trainer and Trainee need to be sufficiently free from over-intrusive anxieties in their private lives. Education is only one part of what each does, and non-professional issues such as finance, health and relationships may compete for attention. The fact that these are outside the formal remit of training does not diminish their power to sap motivational energy.

'Safety' issues

Given adequate 'survival rations', the next set of issues to emerge from a Trainee's early clinical skirmishes centres round the need to be, if not yet proficient, at least a *safe* doctor. Most Trainees are keenly aware of the maxim *'primum non nocere'* – 'above all do no harm'. (And the Trainers of the minority who are not soon become alerted to the primacy of this level of educational concern.) Their prior medical education and hospital experience should have ensured that Trainees have essential clinical knowledge and skills in place, and are competent to deal with urgent or straightforward medical problems. Both Trainers and Trainees, for their own peace of mind, like to check out these assumptions in planned tutorials and 'hot topic' case discussion.

Trainees need to be reassured that, if they acknowledge insecurity in this area, the learning environment can be relied upon to respond helpfully. It is often at this 'safety' stage that Trainees feel most intensely the cognitive dissonance that is to fuel their learning. In order for this to be tolerable, mutative information needs to be quickly and reliably available. The Trainer is looked to as a source of authoritative information, advice and reassurance, backed up if necessary with books and articles from the practice library. Trainers find their support and availability repeatedly put to the test, much as parental rules and boundaries are tested by young children exploring just how secure and trustworthy the adult world will prove. A more didactic teaching style seems appropriate at this stage, "a straight answer to a straight question", in preference to the more heuristic "how shall we find out?" style. Where issues of safety are concerned, points of kairos are usually obvious, and the minimal cues signalling a learning need unmistakeable: "Sorry to interrupt you, but what's the dose of penicillin for a five-year-old?" At this still relatively low order of educational need, what the Trainee requires is the solid information, not practice in tracking it down.

'Confidence' issues

Next up the hierarchy, the equivalent of Maslow's 'belongingness' need, come imperatives heralding a steady growth in the Trainee's confidence. Knowing that safety issues have been addressed and that solid advice is on tap if necessary makes it easier for a Trainee to discover how far he or she can manage without it.

I hope it is not demeaning to compare the trajectory of Traineeship with stages of child development, for the analogy seems to generate some valid perceptions. A child's individuality best flourishes within a stable and mutually benevolent parent/child relationship. The same can be said of the relationship between Trainer and Trainee: stability and mutual benevolence have to be established. In an important sense the Trainer is perceived as *in loco parentis*, and a process of 'bonding' takes place between them, not just at work but perhaps also in the pub, over a meal or on the squash court. This 'parental' projection is temporarily useful in that it establishes at the unconscious level permission for the Trainee to experiment and grow within an ambience of care.

A Trainee learning at the 'confidence' level is making the transition from medicine as seen in hospital to the community version, where illness presents in unfamiliar ways, modified by psychological and social factors and by often bizarre health beliefs. New Trainees' early encounters with the commonplaces of general practice tend to draw responses at the 'safety' level. They seek clear guide-lines, immediate and frequent reassurance. But as confidence is gained they increasingly take the initiative in identifying and rectifying gaps in their knowledge. They learn the diagnostic and therapeutic use of time, and feel increasingly comfortable with putting problems 'on hold'. The corollary of delaying recourse to the Trainer's help is to accept increasing responsibility in the interim. This in turn requires the Trainee to make appropriate use of other members of the practice team without prompting by the Trainer. As a result, he or she becomes accepted as a professional in his or her own right, with a unique and valued contribution to make.

'Recognition' issues

As the Trainee's confidence is regularly tested and confirmed, it becomes internalised as an increasing glow of self-confidence. This is no misplaced cockiness, but rather a hunch, requiring to be verified, that "when all's said and done, I think I've probably got what it takes." This is the equivalent of an 'esteem' need in Maslow's model. Because professional self-confidence is a fragile plant, it needs frequent watering with recognition as a seedling before it can safely be planted out.

An early indication that a Trainee is concerned with 'recognition' issues is when he or she begins to attract a regular following of patients who return with subsequent problems or with other members of their families. Another is an alertness to the existence of patients' 'hidden agenda'. At this 'recognition' stage Trainees become seriously interested in the softer issues of vocational training, such as the dynamics of the doctor/patient relationship or the skills of the consultation, where their own personal style and insights come under scrutiny. They can accept both criticism and praise, because by now they know that the one implies no fundamental weakness and the other imparts no hollow reassurance. They recognise, and can freely discuss, their own personal and professional needs and the ways these impinge on patient care.

It is often an exciting time for Trainer and Trainee when the 'recognition' stage is reached. The Trainee has glimpsed the acme that might be attained, and there is usually a sharp increase in motivational energy at this point. The remainder of the training period seems too brief to cram in everything that might usefully be included. A hunger for fresh ideas and stimulation produces a flurry of interest in, for example, project work and reading. At this point decisions may be made to go on courses to learn new skills or to take the MRCGP exam.

'Self-esteem' issues

If enough other people whose opinions we value indicate that they hold us in high esteem, we are led naturally to the belief that what we have to offer is estimable, and that we ourselves therefore are, as of right and even in the absence of regular confirmation, worthy of that esteem. Self-esteem is not an arrogant feeling for anyone who is ultimately to work unsupervised. On the contrary, it is increasingly necessary for professional survival. As *glaznost* and *perestroika* lap against the walls of medicine's ivory tower, as the gap widens between public expectation and available resources, and as the performance of the GP finds itself ever more minutely scrutinised, belief in the worth of one's work, and of oneself for doing it well, provides an essential bulwark against stagnation or burn-out. So: lower-level issues having been adequately addressed, the nearly-independent Trainee now seeks opportunities to create and confirm a sense of professional self-esteem.

Despite its lofty purpose, it seems inevitable for this to be a period entailing a measure of conflict, overt or covert, between Trainee and Trainer. As the 'self-esteem' phase is entered its psychodynamics tend to be the Oedipal ones of normal adolescence: 'slay the father figure in order to carry off the prize'. To the neophyte, maturity and independence may appear possible only through battle to the symbolic death of the Trainer whose *in loco parentis* role now appears to present an obstacle. Hitherto the Trainer has indeed played a parental role – played it consciously and to good effect; but now their feudal relationship must shift to become one of federacy, of equality with obligations. The bonding necessary in the 'safety', 'confidence' and 'recognition' phases has to some extent to be loosened. Friendship and appreciation may survive, but dependency must not.

As Lipsey observes in his passage on craft apprenticeship quoted in Chapter 1 [2],

> The journeyman is neither child nor adult, neither joyously tied to the mentor nor wholly free. A dark time ensues. Admiration for the mentor is increasingly accompanied by unspoken recognition of his or her shortcomings. . . Furthermore, the mentor himself experiences a subtle change of heart. He cannot help but see that his teaching has failed in many respects; the journeyman is acceptable, perhaps even shows mastery on occasion, but more often seems living proof that the teaching was clumsy.'
>
> [op. cit. pp. 183–4]

In order for both to move on, at this stage Trainee and Trainer need emancipation from their now-redundant parent/child emotional bonding. But simultaneous emancipation, like simultaneous orgasm, is not always the norm. Chagrin and disappointment may briefly befall either party. But it is primarily incumbent on the Trainer to ensure if possible that for the Trainee the experience is a liberating one. The Trainee will be looking for opportunities to establish independence and rectitude, even if initially this means challenging and criticising the fallible mortal the Trainer is ever more clearly perceived to be.

An appropriate analogy would be a rocket on its launch-pad during count-down, still linked to its command tower by umbilical lines carrying information, power and fuel. Once it is fully fuelled the lines will be wrenched away, the gantry swung aside, and lift-off will shortly follow. The 'fuel' taken on at this stage of Traineeship, providing motive force for independent flight, is self-esteem.

Mercifully, the early 'self-esteem' phase is usually less turbulent than its psychodynamics might lead one to suppose. There is by now too great an accumulation of mutual regard, and too adult a control over the transference and counter-transference issues now being enacted. The Oedipal energy is manifest as a growing ability for the Trainee to advise, criticise, challenge, support and educate the Trainer. Knowing his own strengths and limitations, the Trainee increasingly assumes responsibility for devising and implementing his own educational programme. He takes pride in keeping his clinical knowledge and skills up to date, not just to avoid blunders as in the 'safety' phase but because that is what a good doctor should do. As merited self-esteem is acquired, the inevitable uncertainties and failures of practice no longer imply hopeless personal inadequacies. The Trainee discovers that there are more indices of professional competence than the idealised 'doctor as paragon' he may once have envisioned. He can strike a comfortable balance between competing demands of professional and private life. He learns that his own peculiarities of perception and style have a positive contribution to make to his encounters with patients. He begins to understand the diagnostic and therapeutic use of 'himself' in the manner pioneered by Balint [3].

Gradually the emotional ground-rules of the Traineeship become re-worked. If there have been conflictual elements, they are resolved. Independence, though not yet attained, is assured. With this internal certainty the Trainee again feels comfortable with, not oppressed by, the role of learner. The remaining time can be spent looking back in reflection and ahead with confidence.

'Autonomy' issues

The Trainee's successful internalisation of appropriate self-esteem brings to an end the need for a formal educational contribution from the Trainer. Hereafter the Trainer may be welcomed as comrade and confidant; but the protection, stability, reassurance, structure and feed-back he provided during the Traineeship's earlier stages have become relocated as the Trainee's own internal resources. The Trainee is equipped for free flight and now needs just untrammelled space and rights of access to it. He has a fully mature sense of control over his subsequent professional destiny. He feels free to choose and pursue his own clinical interests, and discovers his own ways of enhancing his enjoyment of the rest of his time in the training practice. In motivational terms at least, he is equipped to make a success of the transition from

Trainee to partner. (However, delay in finding a suitable post may cause a Trainee's energy temporarily to regress to lower-order 'survival', 'safety' and 'confidence' issues.)

TEACHING TO THE INNER CURRICULUM

What follows from the idea that educational imperatives form an intrinsic hierarchy? What help is it to believe that Trainees embark on their Traineeships pre-programmed with a sequence of learning stages transcending specific content? Suppose the main features of a training trajectory are indeed pre-mapped; suppose that there is a so-called 'Inner Apprentice' that knows what it needs to know, signals these needs, and indicates whether and when they have been satisfied: so what? Does it help? Aren't such idealisations inevitably swamped by the sheer mass of practical detail to be learned, or rendered academic by the unpredictability of real life? In fact, isn't this Inner Curriculum just a pretty toy for the armchair pundit? It's not a working tool, is it?

Isn't it? Briefly to recapitulate; as training progresses, the focus of educational concentration systematically ascends the hierarchy from bottom to top, from the most basic issues to the most sophisticated, *provided that*:

(1)   lower-level concerns are adequately dealt with before expecting attention to be freed for higher ones; and

(2)   opportunities exist in the educational environment to satisfy successive concerns as the learner becomes ready for them.

The Inner Curriculum and its two requirements, the principles of 'no major holes at the bottom' and 'no barriers to the top', suggest ways for the inner-aware teacher significantly to enhance the efficiency of teaching and learning. If the teacher can identify on any given occasion at what level the Trainee's concern is located, he can pitch the level of his input appropriately. Protection, structure, factual information and clear guidance are needed at the 'security' and 'safety' levels; reassurance and discrete supervision at the 'confidence' level; challenge, encouragement and rigourous pursuit of good practice at the 'recognition' level; insight, interpretation, openness and self-disclosure at the 'self-esteem' level; and unconditional support when 'autonomy' is reached. With a knowledge of the Inner Curriculum, the teacher can more easily tell what aspects of a problem are likely to be taxing the Trainee. He will find it easier to recognise points of kairos in case discussion, reflecting as they do the lowest level of significant inadequacy at the time. He will have a clearer idea of which hierarchical level the Trainee will next be ready for, and (by reading the minimal cues) of when the transition can be expected. This ability to anticipate the next educational need enables the Trainer to prepare a suitable 'expansion space' by offering teaching material and learning opportunities at the right level. He can make a diagnosis in hierarchical terms if the Trainee's learning should appear to stick or regress. The rule of thumb is that 'stagnation at one level indicates residual unattended needs at the previous level down': the remedy then becomes plain.

The trajectory of clinical apprenticeship is of course no smooth curve, nor does skill expand simultaneously in all areas with perfect symmetry. Growth is fitful and, viewed from close up, unpredictable, like the progress of an amoeba putting out pseudopodia in response to invisible local forces. Nevertheless it helps, when we think we might be out of our depth, periodically to touch bottom. The inner-aware teacher can help to keep his contribution aligned with the Trainee's own agenda by periodically asking himself a number of awareness-raising questions:

Awareness-raising questions for teachers

Where are we now on the hierarchy?
How can I tell?
What gaps at what level are being indicated?
How can I tell?
What shall we be concerned with next,
in order to progress?
Are the next level's opportunities available?
If not, how can I create them?
Are there any barriers to attaining the next level?
If so, how can I tell what they are,
and how can they be overcome?

Awareness-raising questions such as these pave the way for some fresh thoughts on the perennial difficulties teachers have with the nature and process of assessment, which we shall return to shortly. In the meantime let me propose to Trainers the exercise of attempting to locate your own Trainee's current place on the hierarchy, using a copy of Figure 9.2 (page 190). Ask him or her to do the same. Then compare and discuss. The exercise will generate answers to most of the questions just posed.

Of carrots and sticks

In Chapter 6 I used the term 'expansion space' to describe the area of educational unexplored territory representing the goals and interests next on the learner's Inner Curriculum. 'Successful completion of one piece of learning' (I suggested) 'releases a readiness for the next. An educational expansion space cannot be arbitrarily imposed, although a skilled teacher may assist in clarifying it. . . Successive expansion spaces follow a hierarchy of priorities, imposing its own inherent sequence and structure on the trajectory of a Traineeship.' Now that we have looked in detail at this hierarchy of priorities, let us re-visit the idea of the expansion space and examine ways of converting the principle into practice. For it could be said that the Trainer's function consists of opening up a succession of expansion spaces for the Trainee, skilfully and appropriately.

Traineeship at its utmost is lived on a threshold, precariously, off balance, with a sense of impending topple into unexplored territory never far away. As we have seen, cognitive dissonance is the official name for that sense of impending topple, and learning is powered by the need to resolve it. Change-inducing cognitive dissonance comes in two types. One, the positively invigorating sort, occurs when we first glimpse the beckoning gap between what we presently are and what we might aspire to become. The other, a more negative and defensive sort, arises when we are brought up short against a different kind of gap, the embarrassing gap between what we had previously liked to think we were and what fresh evidence has painfully revealed us to be. If we liken cognitive dissonance to what it takes to get a mule moving, one is the carrot, and the other the stick.

An example of how the hierarchy can be used as a 'carrot': a Trainee may be functioning effectively at the 'confidence' level, competent in organic medicine and alert to psychological and social modifiers of illness. He may expect the remainder of the Traineeship to consist of 'more of the same' – acquiring greater clinical knowledge, exhibiting keener alertness, and not much else. But there is, as we know, more to general practice than this 'competence at arm's length'. The hierarchy suggests that the next developmental stage will be the 'recognition' level, which includes recognising the diagnostic and therapeutic potential of the doctor's own personality. It can be a useful impetus to learning for the Trainee now to encounter educational material which will introduce this new realm of expertise. He is ready for it, but needs to be shown the 'it' for which he is ready. One of the Balint books would be appropriate, or one of the standard works on the skills of the consultation. If the intervention is well-timed, this material will prove attractive and be eagerly espoused. A thoughtfully-presented glimpse of the next hierarchical expansion space gives the Trainee a specific focus for curiosity.

This is not to deny the role of the 'stick' kind of cognitive dissonance – the revelation of a Trainee's shortcomings – as an educational motivator, but it is a less universal one than is commonly supposed. According to the traditional paradigm, teaching is to be structured and reviewed after formal assessment of curriculum-derived objectives. This mechanistic 'assess before you teach' view of human improvability has saddled Vocational Training with an unfortunate legacy, namely a surplus of sticks and a shortage of carrots [4]. For however tactfully and benevolently it is done, formal assessment is designed to uncover weaknesses, and such exposure cannot but be uncomfortable. Its proponents would say that "discomfort is the price of rigour, and Trainees, though they may not enjoy the process of assessment at the time, will be the better for it in the long run". Any number of articles in the medical education press fervently assert that "if Trainees fail to match up to expectation, they must be assessed all the harder". Much is written about how to make assessment more recipient-friendly, about how to compensate and apologise for the inevitable pain, and about how the agonies of applying the assessment tools hurt the Trainers and Course Organisers far more than the Trainees. Over-reliance on the 'stick' as a method of encouraging diligence, like over-use of the cane in schools, has been responsible for much of the sullen under-achievement lamented by the Course Organisers whose frustrations were documented in Chapter 3. The conventional educational paradigm has simply not inspired today's young Icaruses, nor reliably produced the difference in values and motivation that make the difference. And yet the perceived laissez-faire alternative of shirking assessment entirely seems to promise only anarchy and indiscipline.

How British. How Tom Brown's school-days. And how unnecessary; because once we understand that the imperatives of the learner's own Inner Curriculum can be trusted, and that inner-aligned teaching is efficient teaching, then we are clear to rethink our ideas about assessment and to find more effective ways of using it in the creation of educational expansion spaces.

'Deficiency' and 'growth' motivations

In a later book Maslow drew an important distinction between what he called 'deficiency motivation' and 'growth motivation' [5]. He, of course, was concerned with deeper-going psychological needs than the educational ones which are our present concern: but the parallels are still valuable.

The lower levels of Maslow's hierarchy of needs – 'physiological', 'safety' and in part 'belongingness' – are deficiency needs, in the sense that a person cannot for long remain deficient in them without coming to physical or psychological harm. (Refer back to Figure 9.1 on page 188) Maslow's criteria for a deficiency need [op. cit. p. 22] are that:

(1) Its absence breeds illness;

(2) Its presence prevents illness;

(3) Its restoration cures illness;

(4) In a free choice situation it is pursued by the deprived person in preference to other satisfactions; and

(5) It is no longer of great concern to a healthy person.

Look again at the hierarchy of educational imperatives constituting the Inner Curriculum (Figure 9.2, page 190). Its three lowest levels – 'survival', 'safety' and 'confidence' – fulfil broadly similar criteria. Until deficiencies in these areas have been substantively met a Trainee is at risk, not of illness but of feeling educationally and clinically at sea. A Trainer attempting to interest a deficiency-motivated Trainee in higher-order imperatives is likely to meet resistance or incomprehension. Encountering a complex clinical issue, the deficiency-motivated Trainee will feel most acutely its lower-order challenges, whereas these will not be a problem for the more evolved Trainee whose needs have moved on to the 'recognition' level or beyond.

A Trainee graduating through the lower three levels will no longer be deficient in core clinical skills, but will still not have addressed the remaining higher levels leading to full professional autonomy. He will be safe but nothing special, adequate but unfulfilled, in the same way as someone who in Maslow's terms has physiological and safety needs met but who has not yet experienced the life-enhancing benefits of company, affection, love, appreciation or self-respect. Maslow describes these latter optional extras as 'growth motivations'. They are concerned more with optimising the future than with retrieving the past, proactive rather than reactive. Their equivalents in educational terms are what I have called the 'recognition', self-esteem' and 'autonomy' imperatives. These growth motivations serve to maintain energy for the pursuit of distant and possibly unattainable goals, in contrast to the deficiency needs calling for immediate gratification. Just as ascent of Maslow's hierarchy lifts our motivation from the life-preserving to the life-enhancing, so, as the Inner Curriculum unfolds, the learner's focus of educational concern evolves from the adequacy-ensuring to the career-enhancing.

We are now in a position to understand the origin of the frustrations and disappointments expressed by the Course Organisers and Trainers in Chapter 3, and to know what to do about it.

Hallmarks of excellence (summarised)

Positive response to novelty
'Caritas'
Up-to-date clinical competence
Self-awareness
'Group-ability'
Educability
Motivation
Personal/professional balance
Industry
Communication skills
A sense of mission
Critical ability
Diversity of interests

The 'hallmarks of excellence' we hope to develop in our Trainees (see summary box) consist almost exclusively of values and beliefs that can only be expected of them once they have reached the growth-motivated levels of recognition, self-esteem and autonomy. Unfortunately, most of the educational tools of the trade to date almost exclusively address the deficiency-motivated levels of survival, safety and confidence. We need more carrots, but are stuck with sticks.

"New lamps for old!"

'Trainers in training' emerge from their preparatory courses clutching like a security blanket a package of intellectual tools whose honest intent is to bring order and precision to the process of teaching. With few exceptions these are grounded in the received wisdom that General Practice training can be defined in terms of the Trainee's ability to satisfy a performance-based curriculum of behavioural objectives [6]. This belief has spawned a proliferation of material such as curriculum check-lists, log books, confidence rating scales, and a plethora of formative assessment methods including the doyen of them all, the Manchester Rating Scales [7]. Conventional wisdom says, "Teach only what you can assess, only when you have pre-assessed it, and teach only in ways whose outcome you can measure".

I believe these to be false premises; or rather, incomplete ones. They may provide a suitable programme for robots to teach other robots, and are perfectly appropriate when the educational agenda is (as initially it must be) to remedy deficiencies in knowledge and skills as comprehensively as possible. But they fail to take account of the innate and quirky inquisitiveness that marks us out to be human, not robots. Because curriculum-based teaching defines what needs to be taught by a process of subtraction – by subtracting the learner's measured performance from a quantifiable ideal – its usefulness is restricted to the deficiency motivations of the lower strata of the educational hierarchy, security, safety and confidence. But as Oliver Samuel [8] has reminded us, the General Practice curriculum should be thought of as neither fixed nor finite. It is just as well, therefore, that the native curiosity of the adult learner is also neither fixed nor finite. We have seen how a subliminal awareness of what needs to be learned is already pre-resident in the learner before ever a teacher appears on the scene. And in our study of the Inner Apprentice we have seen what potential we have to learn appropriately and effortlessly once we have noticed the need.

That qualifying clause *"once we have noticed the need"* is crucial, for it redefines the teacher's primary role as assisting the learner to *notice* his current learning needs, as signalled by the various minimal cues we have previously considered. Such traditional teacher activities as telling, measuring, facilitating are in my submission secondary to the raising of non-judgemental awareness.

The habit of telling is hard to break, and the alternative of 'actively noticing' does not come easily. Some puritan ethic survives in the widely-held belief that, to be 'good', learning should be hard work; and teaching, a telling campaign against native ignorance. The awareness-centred teacher sets greater store on noticing than on telling. As we saw in the parallel process of sports coaching, noticing *is* learning; and the process of assisting the learner to notice the cues of his own Inner Apprentice *is* the process of teaching, not just the prelude to it. Awareness-centred teaching requires a higher than usual proportion of the teacher's own attention to be directed outwardly onto minimal cues emitted by the learner, and less of it inwardly trying to work out what ought to be taught. The orthodox educational paradigm promised much, but is now proving a constraining influence. I believe we shall better satisfy the higher aspirations of Trainees (and find teaching more rewarding into the bargain) if we develop greater trust in the power of the awareness-raising question and the use of minimal cues in following the Inner Curriculum.

So I offer an alternative catechism for the awareness-centred teacher:

> *Teach mainly what the Inner Apprentice shows it has noticed the need for. Teach it when the Inner Apprentice indicates it is ready. Teach to the Inner Curriculum in preference to any other. Teach in ways aligned with the Inner Apprentice's preferred learning style, raising non-judgemental awareness and mobilising just-tolerable cognitive dissonance.*

There remains the question of how best to raise non-judgemental awareness at the growth-motivated levels of the educational hierarchy, recognition, self-esteem and autonomy. As the educational focus shifts into the domain of personal attributes and values, teaching needs more than ever to be non-judgemental. The familiar check-lists and rating scales are not equal to the task. The insecurity they generate does not feel safe enough when the Trainee's own personality comes under scrutiny, and for this reason their effectiveness peters out as deficiency needs give way to growth ones. What can we substitute?

Value rating scales

In order to feel comfortable navigating through the growth-motivated regions of the learning trajectory, teachers need some learner-friendly techniques for raising non-judgemental awareness of the value systems and beliefs associated with them. These can often be glimpsed and identified opportunistically in the course of everyday conversation, revealed in value-laden phrases and by minimal behavioural cues such as energy shifts, displacement activities and disturbances of gaze. Behaviour at a grosser level can also make clear statements about current values. A Trainee who is persistently late for surgery, who belittles ancillary staff or who never opens a journal is plainly exhibiting what might euphemistically be termed 'value incongruence'. But it is one thing for a Trainer to suspect value incongruence; it is another to be able to turn such a hunch into an appropriate learning opportunity. I have already suggested that the hierarchy of educational imperatives (Figure 9.2) can be used as a check-list to stimulate formal discussion about higher-order topics. Some more structured approaches might be welcomed, both out of nostalgia for the days of rating scales and out of concern to prevent collusiveness and blind spots arising.

To give them credit, the Manchester Rating Scales do try. They work on the principle of setting out extremes of the quality to be assessed, 'perfect' on the right and 'dreadful' on the left; the assessor rates the Trainee's performance along a ten-point scale between the two. Scale 22, for instance, claims to assess 'Working with colleagues' [9]. The saint on the right *'shows by his/her behaviour toward them that he/she understands the role responsibilities and professionalism of the other members of the primary care team and the practice'*. The villain on the left in contrast *'behaves to colleagues in the practice and the primary care team in a way which suggests that he/she neither understands their role nor respects their professionalism'*.

Ouch!

'Personal development' is rated by Scale 23 [10]. This time the low point of personal development is reached by a doctor who *"does not read medical literature regularly and avoids going to medical meetings. He/she does not always meet consultants on domiciliary visits. He/she is reluctant to be criticized or to take part in evaluation."*

I'll bet! Imagine what it must be like to be rated 2/10 on these scales. Or 5; or even 8. How would you respond? With appreciative curiosity and a renewed sense of purpose? Or with two upthrust fingers?

Values have polarity and intensity; we value A more than B, and to such-and-such a degree. The constructive thing to do when two people have a clash of values is first to identify the nature and extent of the mismatch, and then to discuss it in a non-judgemental and genuinely interested way. Constructive re-evaluation of values, beliefs and priorities is only possible if value incongruence can be identified without overtones of right and wrong, so that neither party is provoked into aggression or defensiveness.

Bearing in mind that values are revealed by the choices we make under pressure, and that they have polarity and intensity, we can proceed as follows.

Take a value-laden issue – say, the merits of a Trainee doing a project – and phrase its two extremes in language which is as far as possible free from bias or implied preference for either (or at least equally loaded in each case). Put the two extremes at opposite ends of a linear analogue scale, and have the two parties, each unseen by the other, indicate their own positions along a continuum between them, as in Figure 9.3.

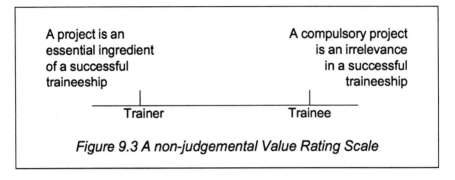

Figure 9.3 A non-judgemental Value Rating Scale

As phrased, neither extreme is obviously 'right and good' or 'wrong and bad'. Someone passionately committed to either can say so without being immediate disparaged by the scale itself. When Trainer and Trainee compare their responses, curiosity not acrimony is aroused. Discussion will generate a series of awareness-raising questions which can be considered without loss of face. In the matter of the Trainee project, *what*, precisely, can't be learned in any other way? *What things* might be more relevant? *What is meant* by 'successful'? *How* essential is 'essential', and *how* compulsory is 'compulsory'?

Figure 9.4 gives another example of how awareness of values can be raised by polarizing two alternatives in a non-judgemental way. Figures 9.5 – 9.7 provide further value rating scales dealing with issues at the 'recognition', 'self-esteem' and 'autonomy' levels respectively. What I have done is take examples from the Inner Curriculum (Figure 9.2) of items at each level and convert them into the format of non-judgemental polarities. They are by no means comprehensive; as with most published

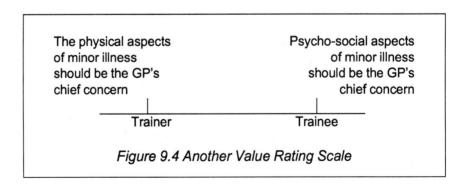

Figure 9.4 Another Value Rating Scale

(Hungry for new ideas)

I like to try out
new ideas for myself
to see if they
might be of value

I like to wait
until new ideas
have proved their value
before trying them

(Hidden agenda)

The physical aspects
of minor illness
should be the GP's
chief concern

Psycho-social aspects
of minor illness
should be the GP's
chief concern

(Confidence not dependent on Trainer's approval)

It's better to be
over-cautious than
over-confident
as a Trainee

To grow in confidence
you have to be
prepared to
take some risks

Figure 9.5 'Recognition' value rating scales

methods of formative assessment they are best used as a template for individual Trainers and workshops to devise their own local variants, to which authorship imparts greater commitment.

Talking about values, beliefs and mission

I suggest that this way of addressing professional values offers a fruitful approach to the problem of 'attitudes', which, as we saw in Chapter 4, have proved such a bugbear that I proposed we should drop the word entirely from the vocabulary of Vocational Training. Value rating scales such as these are quite fun to devise and to use, provided the ensuing dialogue is carried out as far as possible in a similar spirit of non-judgemental interest. Whatever its detailed outcome, the discussion conveys important meta-messages; i.e. the very fact that values can be identified and talked about simultaneously raises significant issues at other levels. 'Clarifying values' indicates to a Trainee that such things are thought relevant to the process of training, and provides a safe

(Can use self in consultations)

A doctor should endeavour
to keep his/her own
feelings out of the
consultation process

A doctor's own feelings
have a significant
contribution to make to
the consultation process

(Personal/professional balance)

There need to be clear
boundaries between a
doctor's on-duty and
off-duty life

A doctor can't expect
always to leave his/her
work behind at the
end of the day

(Tolerates uncertainty)

A problem unsolved
is a problem
insufficiently investigated

Not all problems
have an explanation
or a solution

(Organises own training programme)

The time comes for a
Trainee to take charge
of his/her own
training programme

A Trainer should always
have the final say
over a Trainee's
training programme

(Can challenge Trainer)

A Trainee should always
feel free to criticise
his/her Trainer

It is not a Trainee's
place to criticise
his/her Trainer

(Aware of transference issues)

The relationship between
Trainer and Trainee is
best kept on a purely
professional footing

Awareness of the
relationship between Trainer
and Trainee generates useful
educational insights

Figure 9.6 'Self-esteem' value rating scales

(Takes responsibility for continuing education)

| I believe it is possible for education to change people's personality | I don't think education can really change people's personality |

(Negotiates Trainee/Principal transition)

| If the training has been good, the transition from Trainee to Principal holds few surprises | No matter how good one's training, things are very different as a Principal |

(Sense of overall direction)

| By the end of training, a Trainee should have definite plans for his/her future career | It doesn't matter if a Trainee has no definite career plans by the end of his/her training |

Figure 9.7 'Autonomy' value rating scales

framework for considering topics that might otherwise be found puzzling or contentious. On the other hand, timing and presentation are important. For a Trainer to say, even by implication, "In view of your poor attitude to so-and-so, I propose we do some non-judgemental awareness-raising of your value systems" is itself not non-judgemental. The method should embody the message. It is perfectly possible to 'talk values' without using formal rating scales, by weaving the principle of 'the contrast of unbiased extremes' into ordinary conversation.

As we saw in Chapter 4, values are particularised forms of people's fundamental belief systems. As Trainer and Trainee become clearer about each other's personal and professional values, so their underlying beliefs begin to be discerned. Sensitive discussion can, if the two are willing, lead back in turn to the life events and personal histories that have made them believe the things they do. One of the most powerful awareness-raising methods I have witnessed is an honestly-meant invitation to "Tell me your story." *'Tout comprendre c'est tout pardonner'* runs the French saying – 'to understand everything is to forgive everything'. And to be told the whole story is to understand.

Here is an example, only semi-fictionalised, of how this can work in practice. The members of a Trainers' Workshop have paired off to discuss the attributes they would like their Trainees to develop. Dr A and Dr B agree that one desirable characteristic is that professional and private life should not conflict with each other, but they disagree on what this means. Dr A thinks that if a doctor has any worries in his private life he should keep them to himself, whereas Dr B, on the contrary, considers he should take his partners into his confidence. In the old terminology Dr A does not like Dr B's 'attitude', and vice versa. If they used an assessment tool in the Manchester format, one of them (depending on how the rating scale was phrased) would rate his own attitude as good and the other's as 'needing improvement'. The latter would protest, argue, feel hard done by. Instead Drs A and B draw up the following non-judgemental value rating scale. Any implication of right or wrong is evenly balanced between the two extremes of the scale. Each sounds perfectly tenable, and the scale will allow both A and B to represent their views without significant compromise. They mark their own positions separately as shown:

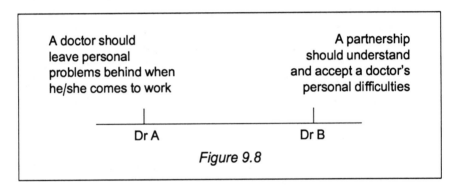

Figure 9.8

Recall that, in the area of values alone, *"Why?"* is an acceptable awareness-raising question. Drs A and B gently unpack the reasons each advances in support of his own position. At first they exchange beliefs. "I believe a partnership is built on trust", says Dr B. "Be that as it may," says A, "I believe it's important to have boundaries." So far, so splendid. But then, recognising that these fine principles are in fact generalisations indicating speech censoring, they ask each other, *"Specifically, what circumstances and experiences have led you to hold that belief?"* It transpires that Dr A has all sorts of domestic worries – aging dependent relatives, rebellious teenage children, over-stretched finances. At home he feels demoralised, ashamed, a failure. He likes to close the front door on his problems when he leaves for work; he prefers the Surgery to be somewhere where people appreciate his strengths and don't remind him of his inadequacies. On the other hand, Dr B's wife has gone off with another man, leaving him with two children under ten. Although he is just about coping, Dr B now has to look to the practice for some of the emotional and practical support his wife had previously supplied. He is lonely. If he is having a bad day at work he needs to be assured of a sympathetic ear without having to explain why. Having exchanged stories, Drs A and B feel closer to each other. They can understand why they have different expectations of their work relationships. Then it dawns on them that at some meta-level they are in fact agreed: each is looking to the practice for partial fulfilment of the needs of the 'doctor as human being'. Values that at first sight seemed irreconcilable stem from a common belief modified only by personal circumstance.

As well as 'talking values', it can be helpful periodically for Trainer and Trainee to 'talk mission'. As the educational focus ascends to growth-motivated levels of the hierarchy so it becomes possible for the Trainee to envision with increasing clarity the goals, hopes and plans to be implemented in the rapidly-approaching future. 'Talking mission' need not be overly sanctimonious, especially if awareness-raising questions are used. "How clearly do you see the way ahead? Are things turning out the way you want them to? Is this what you had imagined your Traineeship would be like? Where does what we are doing at the moment fit into your overall scheme of things? What would you like to concentrate on for the next few days or weeks? How is your idea of a 'good doctor' developing?"

Learning styles analysis

The traditional educational paradigm has more to say on *what to teach* and *how to tell whether it's been learned* than it does on *how to teach* it. Choice of an appropriate teaching and learning format is left to the skilled discretion of the Trainer. And while in this book I have suggested that teachers can and should become more responsive to the agenda-setting, timing and formatting cues emitted by their pupils, I have not considered in detail the differences in preferred learning style that undoubtedly exist between individual learners. Honey and Mumford have developed a most helpful approach to this topic, which I commend to Trainers [11]. They identify four stages in the process of incorporating new mutative information. All are necessary, but individuals tend to be better at some than at others. The invitation to teachers and learners is first to identify and then to address those phases which they are weakest in.

Honey and Mumford distinguish four successive stages during the learner's transit of a given learning opportunity.

(1) A stage of exposure to new ideas and new experiences: people with a stimulus-hunger for novelty are described as *'activists'*.

(2) A stage of reflection, when all angles and implications are considered, and as much relevant data as possible collected: people who like to do this thoroughly are termed *'reflectors'*.

(3) A stage where new material is intellectually integrated with and incorporated into what was previously known, so that a new cognitive understanding can be logically built up: people for whom this is a priority are *'theorists'*.

(4) A stage of trying out the newly-acquired knowledge in practice, to see how it works out in real life: people for whom 'the proof of the pudding is in the eating' and who reserve judgement until they can put new ideas to the practical test are *'pragmatists'*.

Honey and Mumford have devised their Learning Styles Questionnaire (LSQ) to help people identify the type and degree of their preferences. The LSQ contains 80 statements, which you tick if you agree with, of the type 'I tend to be a perfectionist' or 'In discussions I like to get straight to the point'. A marking schedule then tells you how much of a pragmatist, theorist, reflector or activist you are in your preferred learning style. It helps for a Trainer and Trainee to know their own and each other's tendencies, so that collusiveness and blind-spots can be predicted and overcome. Like value rating scales, the LSQ is an awareness-raising tool useful in its own right and also as a means of bringing into the open stylistic mismatches which might otherwise disrupt and distort the teaching relationship. The contact address for obtaining LSQ material is given in this chapter's references [11].

Inner-aligned teaching in context

Figure 9.9 is an attempt to articulate the material discussed in this book into an overall approach to Vocational Training which is *inner-aligned*, i.e. more synergistic with the learner's intrinsic learning needs and methods. The left-hand side of the diagram shows how beliefs and value systems provide a slowly evolving link between a person's past – his or her cultural background and life events – and the future he or she endeavours through education to create. On the right is the array of ideas and interventions available to the awareness-centred teacher, showing stages and processes in professional growth to which they can be applied.

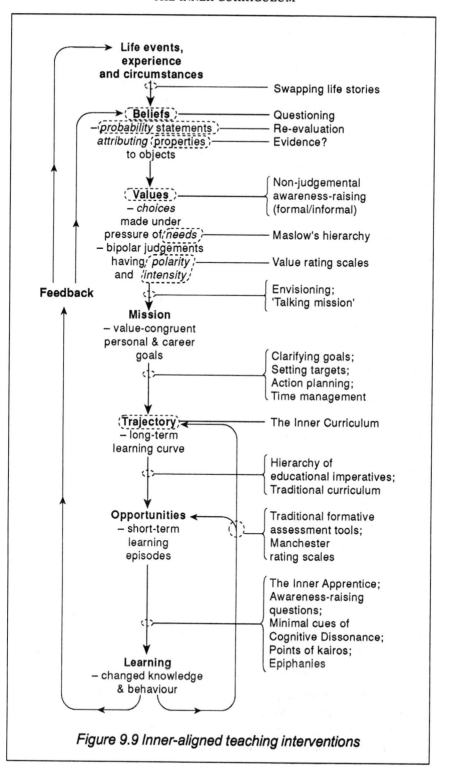

Figure 9.9 Inner-aligned teaching interventions

It has been a central thesis of this book that adult vocational education derives most of its energy and structure and many of its daily points of interest from the learner's pre-resident learning resources. Inner-aligned teaching therefore proceeds by cultivating an educational environment within which these intrinsic forces, dubbed the Inner Apprentice, are freely released to follow their own course. The essential principle is for the teacher constantly to be raising and updating the learner's conscious non-judgemental awareness of the way things currently are. Periodically this active noticing results in educationally useful cognitive dissonance. The learner is motivated to relieve this 'psychic irritation'; it is the teacher's responsibility to ensure that relief takes the form of appropriate learning. If it does, the reward is a release of energy lifting the focus of attention to higher levels of the Inner Curriculum.

Medical teachers still wedded to the belief that assessment is the power-house of effective learning may protest that there seems no place in this scheme of things for 'proper' formative assessment, except a grudgingly conceded role in meeting deficiency needs towards the bottom of the educational hierarchy. On the contrary: assessment is all-pervading. It depends, as Professor Joad used to say on *The Brains Trust*, on what you mean by assessment. If you mean an episodic process, carried out at arbitrary intervals as a set-piece exercise, and intended to provide a Trainee with feedback on his not-necessarily-recent performance and to assist a Trainer to plan his teaching in the not-necessarily-immediate future, then no – that kind of assessment is not very helpful. I was once on a five-day course on clinical hypnosis presented by Steve and Carol Lankton in Florida. Towards the end of the final day someone asked when we would get to fill out the post-course assessment forms. "Whenever you like," said Steve, " – but how will you know when you've stopped learning?"

If on the other hand we think of assessment not as a process but as a frame of mind, then I'll be first among its champions. Assessment is the frame of mind that is untiringly interested in making conscious whatever the Trainee is just on the threshold of learning. Assessment is the frame of mind that values relevance and good timing in teaching. Assessment is the frame of mind that keeps three questions hovering in the teacher's thoughts – *"How can I help this person become fully aware of what matters most right now? What does matter most right now? And how can I tell?"*

Probably the most important and sensitive assessment tool is the teacher's own power of attention. Watch a skilled cardiologist assessing a patient's heart murmur: his skill resides not in which brand of stethoscope he uses, but rather in the knowledge of where to place it most efficiently in order to obtain the highest-grade clinical information. The inner-aware teacher practises placing his own attention with the same precision on the learner's minimal cues, and is similarly rewarded with the highest-grade educational information.

> *Assess* before *you teach, if you need to.*
> *Assess* after *you teach, if you need to.*
> *Assess* while *you teach,* because *you need to.*

THE LEGACY OF SOCRATES

We have come a long way – or have we? – in the twenty-five centuries since Chapter 1, when we eavesdropped on Socrates as he sat upon his wall, irascible and eccentric, mercilessly educating anyone who dared engage him in dialectic on the subject of how to seek personal excellence. As a public figure Socrates was, literally, fatally short on tact. He was condemned for daring to suggest that although men were improvable, those in power were not necessarily the ones who had bothered over-much about improving themselves. We should today find plenty to criticise about Socrates' teaching skills. He appears to have specialised in the one-off tutorial; few of his interlocutors had sufficient stamina or masochism to come back for more. Possibly Socrates himself was unsure how to string together a series of insights into the larger trajectory we now know to be important. He clearly knew that the important civilised qualities lay in the realms of values and beliefs; and he knew how to turn a pitiless spotlight onto attitudes normally left to lurk undisturbed in the gloom of the psyche. But even if Socrates was indeed the 'midwife to ideas' he professed to be, he was certainly no neonatal paediatrician, proving consistently ineffectual at nurturing premature and fragile insights into a sturdy maturity. He seemed insensitive to the minimal cues that marked a pupil's transition from interest to indignation, from a longing for enlightenment to a longing merely for escape.

We can nevertheless appreciate Socrates' strengths. He was the implacable enemy of teachers who taught to a formula, or who taught whatever passing fads pleased their paymasters, or who taught in order to exert control over others. He knew that, if we want to learn, we must first experience our own ignorance. Above all, he recognised that fundamental knowledge of what is good lies pre-resident in all people, and that systematic questioning is the way to release it. These are valuable legacies.

We are legatees also of the great medieval institution of apprenticeship. Rigours and ritual notwithstanding, to be apprentice and journeyman to a master-craftsman was a substantial privilege. Even though some of its formal trappings may have fallen away, apprenticeship remains pre-eminent as a model for the process and psychodynamics of contemporary Vocational Training. As Lipsey's account shows, the apprenticeship system was more than a vehicle for imparting a core curriculum of knowledge and practical skills. Of no less value was the process of psychological maturation occurring within, and by virtue of, a close relationship with a personal mentor. If the words 'Trainer' and 'Trainee' were by proclamation to be stricken from the vocabulary, I should propose as substitutes 'mentor' and 'apprentice'.

I appear to be pleading nostalgically for a return to much older ways of doing things; and to some extent I am. The infra-structure and micro-structure of curriculum-based teaching, for all its initially promising shiny new gloss, is beginning to look a little tarnished and inadequate. The curriculum-based educational paradigm, I believe, is in any case something of a myth: not a myth in the sense of an untruth or a figment of the imagination, but a mythological system of beliefs whose truth is symbolic, stylised and over-simplified in order to imply universality and to inspire awe. We are just not so simple as the paradigm requires us to suppose.

Miller Mair, a clinical psychologist and psychotherapist in Dumfries, has written trenchantly of the ease with which too slavish an adherence to dogmas and paradigms can crowd out the human sensitivity that real growth is predicated upon [12]. Although in these quotations he is writing about therapy, his critique applies equally well to a style of teaching that is too curriculum-based and assessment-centred.

> Put simply, I believe that intimate knowledge is likely to teach us more than distant knowledge. Personal knowledge is likely to change us more than impersonal knowledge. Knowledge gained with our eyes, ears and imaginations wide open is likely to be more valuable than that acquired when we are conceptually and procedurally blindfolded. . . Knowledge acquired through the patient process by which the questioner takes time to be trusted and to show care for the answerer is likely to be more significant than that gained by the 'hit and run' merchant who only wants to make a quick psychological 'buck'. . . . At present (we are) both grounded *on* and grounded *by* too lumbering an adherence to formal procedures (and by too rigid an insistence on) defining reliable knowledge as that which emanates from these set-piece engagements with a sawn-up world.
>
> [op. cit. pp. 2–3]

If the spirit of Socrates and the ghosts of the medieval apprentice-masters are able to divert us from too many 'set-piece engagements with a sawn-up world', let us welcome them. They remind us (if we need to be reminded) that teaching, before it is lists and strategies, is above all a special way of being with another person. To find a way of being like Socrates, but without the vainglory; to find a way of being like the medieval craftsmen, offering our apprentices mastery but without the misery – these are heroic tasks for today's teachers. Surely our shoulders will fit the mantle bequeathed to us? To be *that* kind of hero is no ignoble goal.

References and Bibliography

CHAPTER 1 – ON APPRENTICESHIP

1. Illich, I. (1976) *Limits to Medicine. Medical Nemesis: The Expropriation of Health.* (London: Marion Boyars). Summarised in its opening sentence: 'The medical establishment has become a major threat to health.' Also: (1977) *Disabling Professions.* (London: Marion Boyars). 'Informed choice requires that we examine the specific role of the professions in determining who got what from whom and why.'

2. See, for example:

    Bandler, R. and Grinder, J. (1975) *Patterns of the Hypnotic Techniques of Milton H. Erickson, M.D.* (Cupertino, California: Meta Publications). 'Transformational grammarians have built an explicit representation of the intuitions which people demonstrate when communicating and understanding natural language.'

    Also, same authors; (1975) *The Structure of Magic (I).* (Palo Alto, California; Science and Behavior Books).

3. Schloegl, I. (1977) *The Zen Way.* (London: Sheldon Press).

4. Stott, N.C.H. and Davis, R.H. (1979) The exceptional potential in each primary care consultation. *J. R. Coll. Gen. Pract.*, 29, 201–5.

5. Neighbour, R.H. (1987) *The Inner Consultation.* (Lancaster: MTP Press).

6. Byrne, P.S. and Long, B.E.L. (1976) *Doctors Talking to Patients.* (London: HMSO).

7. Pendleton, D., Schofield, T., Tate, P. and Havelock, P. (1984) *The Consultation: an Approach to Learning and Teaching.* (Oxford: Oxford University Press).

8. Plato, trans. Guthrie, W.K.C. (1956) *Protagoras and Meno.* (London: Penguin Books). The *Meno* is a particularly helpful half-hour's read for aspiring Trainers.

9. Both the mathematical processes and the educational theories are more fully described in Guthrie, *op. cit.* pp. 107–114.

10. Working Party of the Royal College of General Practitioners. (1972) *The Future General Practitioner: Learning and Teaching.* (London: British Medical Journal).

11. Shaffer, P. (1973) *Equus.* (London: Andre Deutsch).

12. Plato, trans. Hamilton, W. (1973) *Phaedrus.* (London: Penguin Books). The passage quoted is from page 97.

13. Plato, trans. Lee, D. (1955) *The Republic.* (London: Penguin Books).

14. Lipsey, R. (1988) *An Art Of Our Own: the Spiritual in Twentieth Century Art.* (Boston, Massachusetts: Shambhala Publications). A stunning and inspirational book. Whatever one's interest in art, to open it is to find oneself in a gallery of ideas illumined with shafts of brilliant insight.

15. Hemery, D. (1986) *The Pursuit of Sporting Excellence: a Study of Sport's Highest Achievers.* (Champaign, Illinois: Human Kinetics Books). An authoritative and fascinating study by one of England's great athletes. Chapter 8, Coach-Athlete Relationship, and Chapter 13, Creativity, Visualization and Imagery, are of particular interest to Vocational Trainers.

CHAPTER 2 – THE STORY OF DAEDALUS AND ICARUS

1. See reference 10, Chapter 1.

2. One example is the Trainee-held loose-leaf 'log book' devised and used by the North West Thames Region, British Postgraduate Medical Federation. Enquiries should be addressed to: The Regional Adviser's Office, North West Thames Region, Hammersmith Hospital, Ducane Road, London W12 0HS.

3. Berne, E. (1966) *Games People Play.* (London: Andre Deutsch).

4. Graves, R. (1955) *The Greek Myths.* (London, Penguin Books).

5. Neighbour, R.H. (1990) Icarus and Daedalus: myths, methods and motivation in vocational training; Paper I, The Icarus Factor. *Postgraduate Education for General Practice*, 1, 30–37.

6. Cox, M. and Theilgaard, A. (1987) *Mutative Metaphors in Psychotherapy: the Aeolian Mode.* (London: Tavistock Publications). Like the Lipsey book (ref. 1.14), an unexpected motherlode of insight, despite its daunting title. The authors bring together wide-ranging material from literature to neurophysiology in support of their premise; namely, that psychotherapists do well to let their listening minds resonate to metaphor and allegory in the stories their patients tell them.

7. Bachelard, G. (1969) *The Poetics of Space.* (Boston: Beacon Press).

CHAPTER 3 – THE HALLMARKS OF EXCELLENCE

1. Hickman, Craig R. and Silva, Michael A. (1985) *Creating Excellence: Managing Corporate Culture, Strategy & Change in the New Age.* (London: Unwin Paperbacks).

2. Garfield, C. (1986) *Peak Performers: The New Heroes in Business.* (London: Hutchinson Business).

3. Maslow, Abraham H. (1970) *Motivation and Personality*, 2nd edn. (New York: Harper & Row).

4. "The difference that makes the difference": a favourite phrase of the anthropologist Gregory Bateson, often quoted by him in books and conversation.

CHAPTER 4 – THE DIFFERENCE THAT MAKES THE DIFFERENCE

1. "Not everything that counts can be counted ..." An epigram attributed to Sir George Pickering, and, so the story goes, kept by Albert Einstein permanently chalked on his blackboard at Princeton.

2. Cotgrove, Stephen F. (1982) *Catastrophe or Cornucopia: The Environment, Politics and the Future.* (Chichester: Wiley).

3. See reference 2, Chapter 3, page 271.

4. Bohm, D. and Rossi, E. (1988) Beyond relativity and quantum theory: an interview with David Bohm. *Psychological Perspectives*, vol. 19, no. 1, pp. 25–43. (Los Angeles: C. J. Jung Institute of Los Angeles).

CHAPTER 5 – THE INNER APPRENTICE

1. Gallwey, W. Timothy (1975) *The Inner Game of Tennis.* (London: Jonathan Cape). Also: (1981) *The Inner Game of Golf.* (London: Jonathan Cape).

2. I am indebted to the skill and friendship of Alan Fine in showing me at first hand the process of awareness-centred sports coaching. For information on the application of this approach in business as well as in sport, contact Alan Fine at: InsideOut Development Ltd., 6 Adam & Eve Mews, Kensington, London W8 6UJ.

3. See reference 6, Chapter 2.

4. Conrad, Barbara (1990) The Obligatory Sex Scene, in: *The Complete Guide to Writing Fiction*, Chapter 16, page 178. (Cincinnati, Ohio: Writer's Digest Books).

CHAPTER 6 – HOW THE INNER APPRENTICE LEARNS

1. Festinger, L. (1957) *A Theory of Cognitive Dissonance.* (Evanstown, Illinois: Row, Peterson).

2. For a clear account of Cognitive Dissonance and its relevance to medical topics such as placebos, hypnosis and psychosomatic illness, see:

   Totman, R. (1979) *Social Causes of Illness.* (London: Souvenir Press).

3. Forster, E. M. (1910) *Howards End.* Available in Penguin Classics (London: Penguin Books). Quoted passage from Chapter 4.

4. Forster, E. M. (1924) *A Passage to India.* Available in Penguin Classics (London: Penguin Books). Quoted passage from Chapters 15 and 16.

CHAPTER 7 – MINIMAL CUES

1. Dickinson, E. (c.1861) In *A Choice of Emily Dickinson's Verse*, selected by Ted Hughes (1968) (London: Faber and Faber).

2. Neighbour, R.H. (1987) *The Inner Consultation.* (Lancaster: MTP Press).

CHAPTER 8 – THE POINT OF KAIROS

1. See reference 6, Chapter 2.

2. Hammer, E.F. (1968) *Use of Interpretation in Treatment.* (New York: Grune & Stratton).

3. Freud, S. (1900) *The Interpretation of Dreams.* Standard Edn. Vols. 4 and 5. (London: Hogarth Press and the Institute of Psychoanalysis).

4. Heider, J. (1985) *The Tao of Leadership: Leadership Strategies for a New Age.* (New York: Bantam Books).

CHAPTER 9 – THE INNER CURRICULUM

1. See reference 3, Chapter 3. 1st edn. (1954).

   Also: Maslow, Abraham H. (1976) *Religions, Values, and Peak-Experiences.* (Harmondsworth, Middlesex: Penguin Books).

2. See reference 14, Chapter 1.

3. Balint, M. (1971) *The Doctor, His Patient and The Illness.* 2nd edn.. (London: Pitman Medical).

4. Billington, T. (1990) Carrot or stick? How to get the best out of a trainee. *Postgraduate Education for General Practice*, 1, 38-41.

5. Maslow, Abraham H. (1968) *Toward a Psychology of Being.* 2nd edition. (New York: D. Van Nostrand Company).

6. See, for example, reference 10, Chapter 1.

   Also: Hall, M. S. (Ed.) (1989) *A GP Training Handbook.* 2nd edn.. (Oxford: Blackwell Scientific Publications).

7. Centre for Primary Care Research, Department of General Practice, University of Manchester. (1988) *Rating Scales for Vocational Training in General Practice.* Occasional Paper 40. (London: Royal College of General Practitioners).

8. Samuel, O. (1990) *Towards a Curriculum for General Practice Training.* Occasional paper 44. (London: Royal College of General Practitioners).

9. See reference 7, Chapter 9, page 24.

10. Op. cit. page 25.

11. Honey, P. and Mumford, A. (1986) *The Manual of Learning Styles.* 2nd edn.. Published and distributed by: Peter Honey, Ardingly House, 10 Linden Avenue, Maidenhead, Berkshire SL6 6HB.

12. Mair, M. (1989) *Between Psychology and Psychotherapy: A Poetics of Experience.* (London: Routledge).